12.00

ESCAPE YOUR WEIGHT

ALSO BY EDWARD JACKOWSKI, Ph.D.

Escape Your Shape

Hold It! You're Exercising Wrong.

ESCAPE

SELECT YOUR OWN PERSONAL OPTION FOR LOOKING AND FEELING FABULOUS

Thomas Dunne Books · *St. Martin's Press* ≋ *New York*

Your Weight

HOW TO WIN AT WEIGHT LOSS

EDWARD JACKOWSKI, Ph.D.

THOMAS DUNNE BOOKS.
An imprint of St. Martin's Press.

www.stmartins.com

Designed by Fritz Metsch

ISBN 0-312-31199-0

FIRST EDITION: JANUARY 2004

10 9 8 7 6 5 4 3 2 1

Contents

50 Incentives to Lose Weight and Get Fit

- It's good for you.

- You'll live longer.

- You'll live a more productive life while living longer.

- You'll be healthier.

- You'll possess a stronger immune system.

- You'll lower your chances of catching the common cold.

- You'll lower your chances of developing various forms of cancer.

- You'll recover faster from injuries or surgery.

- You'll be stronger as you become older, and if you fall you won't fracture your hips or legs as easily.

- You'll combat diabetes, osteoporosis, and many other ailments that would normally debilitate you.

- You'll have a better sex life.

- You'll have more confidence.

- You'll possess better self-esteem and a more positive body image.

- You'll be more comfortable naked.

- You'll get naked.

- You'll be more active.

- You'll choose more activity-type hobbies.

- You'll better perform your favorite sport or leisure activity.

- You'll enjoy your favorite sport or leisure activity more.

- You'll pick more active and healthier friends.

- You'll no longer be lazy.

- You'll be more disciplined in every facet of your life.

- You'll manage your stress more effectively.

- You'll be able to play more with both your children and grandchildren.

- You'll live long enough to have grandchildren.

- You'll feel better in public.

- You'll actually be more social and go out in public.

- You'll no longer hear people snickering behind your back, aghast about how "big" you are.

- You'll have more job opportunities.

- You'll make more money.

- You'll have more control in every aspect of your life.

- You'll greatly increase your chances of meeting a lifetime partner.

- You'll be able to share things with your partner (such as working out together).

- You'll possess more mental focus.

- You'll accomplish more with your life.

- You'll overcome obstacles and hurdles and all the curveballs that life throws at you.

- You'll spend less time sitting on your butt.

- You'll earn and appreciate it when you do relax and choose to do nothing.

- You'll have less guilt when you have a "bad" eating day.

- You'll have far fewer "bad" eating days.

- You'll be able to eat and drink whatever you desire—within moderation of course.

- You'll never have to worry about gaining weight if you have a glass of fine wine or your favorite food or an occasional dessert.

- You'll be happier and smile more often.

- You'll spend less time and money on a therapist and be less depressed.

- You'll be able to put away that extra money saved.

- You'll have more energy and experience fewer mood swings.

- You'll have more focus and be able to persevere through any dilemma.

- You'll be more ambitious.

- You'll be much better at golf, tennis, or any other sport you enjoy.

- You'll love life.

- You'll love yourself.

TO BE SUCCESSFUL AT LOSING

AND MAINTAINING WEIGHT

LOSS, I MUST ACCEPT THE FACT

THAT IT CAN *ONLY* BE ACHIEVED

BY EATING SENSIBLY AND EX-

ERCISING REGULARLY; OTHER-

WISE, I WILL *NEVER* REALIZE

MY GOAL OF LOOKING,

FEELING, AND FUNCTIONING AT

MY BEST.

Introduction

How smart would your child be if you only read to him/her once a week for a short while? How about studying a new language a few times a month? What if you baked a cake and didn't have all the ingredients; would it come out edible? To be good at fitness, like anything else in life, requires regularity and an exact process; otherwise you will fall way short of realizing your goals.

Wait a minute; I thought this book was about weight loss? It is; relax; I am just alerting you as to the process necessary to lose and maintain weight loss. The first thing you must realize and *accept* is that success at losing and keeping weight off your body can only be achieved by exercising regularly and properly *plus* eating sensibly. There is no other way. There is no negotiating. Oh, and by the way, you will have to do these two things: work out and eat properly, for the rest of your life, not just for a month or two or until you shed some excess weight.

Throughout this book and beyond, you will read things that are completely opposite what you have read or have heard elsewhere. Therefore, when I explain a certain point or emphasize a particular subject I will always try to support it with scientific or medical data and/or logic, so that you, the reader, can intelligently challenge all the fallacies out there circulating, cluttering your mind and confusing you no end. I am simply the messenger, more precisely, your messenger, whose function is to educate and motivate you and make you aware of what is necessary to master permanent weight loss. You might not like or agree with some of the things you'll see and learn in this book, but too bad. I need to tell you

Escape Route #1: In short, you have to *earn* the right to look and feel great just as you have earned the right to be good at your job!

and expose you to the pitfalls and the dos and don'ts that either you have already encountered or are silly attempts you are contemplating in order to lose weight. *Everything* that is depicted in this book is medically and scientifically proven. I do not speak or write on what I "think" is accurate or what I'm emotionally tied to. I speak the truth, and that's important for you, the reader, to know and understand so that you have a certain comfort factor when you judge the validity and source of information as you start your quest to lose weight.

One of the first things I will teach you is that fitness, weight management, nutrition, health, energy, being productive, and being active are all synonymous and one and the same. So when I use such phrases as *becoming more fit* or *the importance of being active* or *eating sensibly,* I always mean all of the above. To better understand this point, there are certain elements, protocol, and a process vital to your physically being the best you can be.

And one of the biggest mistakes a lot of people make toward becoming more fit is actually thinking that they can become fit by being more active.

What is the function and purpose of being fit? Well, aside from good health, it's to enjoy all the wonderful things that life has to offer: hiking, walking, golf, tennis, skiing, gardening, canoeing, yard work, or however you wish to move your body, occupy your mind, and enjoy yourself.

Over the last twenty years of teaching lifestyle management, I have heard and seen practically every excuse as to why someone cannot lose weight. The reality of the situation is that it boils down to two main reasons that 99 percent of these people have failed at weight loss: (1) the process or methods selected were flawed, or (2) it wasn't important enough or a big enough priority for them to take the necessary steps in order to be successful. The other 1 percent failed because of truly medical-related and valid reasons. That being said, I have always maintained that it's easier to go to work five days a week for eight hours than it is to work out five days a week for one hour. Think about how ridiculous yet true this is. In fact, only 10 percent of the entire population exercise only two or three times per week 40/52 weeks. Now you can clearly see why nearly 75 percent of our population are either clinically obese and/or overweight *and* out of shape. Actually, I should put you at ease here. The exercise part is really quite simple and not difficult at all. It's the planning, organization, and fitting proper fitness into your everyday lifestyle coupled with performing the correct exercises to reach your goals that presents the challenge for most.

It's time for me to introduce myself to you. My name is Dr. Edward

Escape Route #2: You cannot become fit by being more active; you can only be more active by becoming fit.

Jackowski. I am an expert at making *proper* fitness part of anyone's lifestyle despite any constraint. I am a businessman in the business of fitness, not a fitness guy trying his hand at business. I am also one of the few people in the fitness industry whose philosophy has not changed since I have entered this field over twenty years ago. What has changed for the better is my ability to communicate my expertise to you, the knowledge I've gained on maximizing hard-earned time in search of losing weight, becoming and staying fit for the rest of your life.

Aside from being the CEO of one of America's largest and most successful one-on-one motivational and fitness companies, I have devoted over half my life to helping individuals from all walks of life to be their best, using fitness as a catalyst to help overcome any curveball that life may throw at them. In addition, I answer each and every E-mail that comes across my desk along with taking every phone call from anyone trying to reach out for help, day in and day out. I don't hang out in a gym all day, pop protein pills, or lift weights like your typical jock. In many ways, I am just like you, a hardworking individual who needs to prioritize and organize my daily activities in order to eat sensibly and exercise regularly. And if I overeat or skip my workouts, guess what? I actually gain weight. The difference, though, is that I don't allow myself to get off track for too long, because I have built in certain incentives and motivational tools that have allowed me to devise the most powerful fitness regimen in existence today, which permits me to lose a few pounds just as easily as gaining a few pounds—*without* starving myself or taking other extreme measures to get back on track.

This book is about sharing winning formulas with you that I have gleaned from people just like you so that you, too, can control your own destiny when it comes to weight management. And, you will learn, too, that when you yourself get off track, you shall go back to that winning formula—by watching *your* food intake and exercising with a purpose. No matter how well I eat, I still don't feel as good as when I exercise. The synergy, of course, of both eating well and exercising consistently is the ultimate prize.

One of the most amazing things I encounter when I sit down with an individual to discuss his/her lifestyle, diet, and exercise habits is that *nearly* everyone is willing to try any means to try to lose weight, and most of these futile attempts are so mind-boggling to me that I cannot understand how a successful, rational person would even contemplate any of these in the first place! I always find it astonishing that anyone would attempt to go on a crash diet for weeks on end to lose weight rather than cut his/her food intake by a third and exercise a few days per week,

> *Escape Route #3:* A great fitness program can make up for a poor diet, but a great diet can *never* make up for lack of a proper fitness program.

allowing him/her to actually lose *more* weight, without the mental and physical stress they put on their systems. Believe me, I tell him/her, if you have the willpower to starve yourself, then you certainly have the mental fortitude to *not* starve yourself and work out a few days per week. Aside from the health consequences from "dieting," the human body cannot maintain the denial for long periods of time of certain nutrients our bodies and minds crave. And I don't care how much willpower you think you have, when the body says feed me, believe me, you will eat, and because you are in such deficit, you will inevitably overeat.

Everyone is always looking for the shortcut in life. Be it diet, exercise, work, making money, et cetera, we all, for the most part, want instant gratification. Well, trust me, Susan or Robert, you didn't gain 50 pounds in three months, so what makes you think you can lose it in a few short months?

You want to know a secret? Here's a tip: the shortcut to losing and maintaining weight loss is *stop overeating* and *start overexercising*! You know it's funny, in all the years of helping people achieve weight loss and fitness, I *never* once met an individual who ate sensibly and exercised properly and consistently who *did not* lose weight, improve his/her health, increase his/her fitness level, and look great. And the *only* people who didn't achieve their weight-loss and other fitness-related goals were what I call the Burger Kings: they did it "their way," not the correct way.

The theme of this book is thinking inside the box. Typically, we almost always see or hear the exact opposite expression: "You need to think outside the box." Well, that may be good for finance or if you want to be an entrepreneur, but when it comes to fitness and weight loss it will hurt you. What I mean by "thinking inside the box" is that fitness and weight loss is a process, which requires certain and exact dos and don'ts. I am not interested in what you think will work, what your partner thinks, or what your "trainer" says. Why? Because quite simply, if these people knew anything about what it takes for you to look and feel your best, you wouldn't be 10, 20, 50, or more pounds overweight and you would be assisting them in writing this book.

We all want the z in life, but few are willing to go *a, b, c, d, e, f, g, h, i, j, k, l, m, n, o, p, q, r, s, t, u, v, w, x, y, z*. This book is about following this exact order, not skipping from *A* to *K*, *N* to *V*, et cetera. This is what I mean by thinking "inside the box." No jumping ahead or varying is allowed.

I have worked my tail off for 20 years mastering this system, and believe me, if there was another way or a simple pill we could take to look and feel our best, I wouldn't be wasting my time or your time. Just an

FYI: I have garnered over 10,000 letters/testimonials over the years from people of all walks of life who were smart enough to have listened to my advice by *only* thinking inside the box and thus have been successful meeting their fitness and weight-loss goals. You are not a rat or an experiment. Nor do I "think" this will work. It works, but you have to work at being honest with yourself and sticking to the plan without *any* deviations. And it doesn't matter whether you have 10 pounds to lose or 100 pounds to lose; the process is still the same. What is different is the time element to achieve your weight-loss and fitness goals. In fact, it's easier for an overweight individual to lose weight than it is for someone who is underweight to try to gain or keep weight on. You know why? Because in order for that underweight person to gain weight (and look good of course), that person needs to eat so many times and exercise a lot more than you who are overweight. Thus there are more chances that he/she will make more mistakes.

That's why I am such a big proponent of exercise as being the *main* ingredient in treating weight loss. Aside from the fact that proper exercise raises your Basal Metabolic Rate (known as your BMR), we only need to perform fitness three to five times per week in order to lose weight and look and feel great. However, we eat at least three to five times a day.

When you look at it from a statistical point of view and on a weekly basis, we only need to exercise 3–5 times out of seven days, compared to eating 21–35 times out of seven days. The odds of eating poorly during one week are *far* greater than the odds of being and making fitness a consistent part of that same week.

My goal is to get you to a point where you can achieve five days of eating well combined with four or five days of exercising properly. When you can achieve this, not for merely a week here and there, then and only then will you reach self-actualization and achieve that nirvana of looking and feeling your best!

This book is about efficiency and effectiveness. I don't want you to become obsessed and focus on losing weight. I want you to focus on whatever it takes to exercise three to five days per week coupled with eating sensibly five days per week on a weekly basis. That's what you need to be obsessed with. And if, by the way, you are clever enough to focus on these two elements you will undoubtedly achieve permanent weight loss.

This one is one of my favorites: "Edward, I want to go on a diet before I start exercising and I promise to call you in a month or two after I have lost some weight." Well, I am still waiting for that call. This is clearly someone who is not thinking inside the box.

Escape Route #7: You need to approach and look at fitness and weight loss on a weekly basis rather than on a daily basis.

Escape Route #8: Exercise is the most effective way of forming better eating habits; dieting however, cannot and does not act as a catalyst for starting an exercise program. The reason is that when we severely diet we have very low energy-levels and the thought of moving or exercising is so exhausting both mentally and physically.

I would say that this is perhaps the biggest faux pas that people make when embarking on a weight-loss program. Don't get trapped into this facade. Remember to *only* think "inside the box" at all times.

It's not entirely your fault. The majority of magazines, books, or infomercials all have the same message: Lose weight by magical pills, diets that promise fast results, and unfounded exercise claims that all you need to do is exercise eight minutes a day and you will lose weight and look great. Now ask yourself this simple question; if all we needed to do was take a pill or walk a bit or eliminate carbohydrates from our diet, then why are we as fat as we are?

The answer is that losing weight, becoming fit, and looking our best can only be achieved by eating properly and exercising correctly and consistently. Now that, my friend, is a claim that I can definitely substantiate. Yet we as Americans, and, for that matter, people worldwide, are taking the ingredients that make up the medical and scientific formula for weight loss and picking and choosing certain elements out of this formula and concocting our own mixture. We don't follow directions and are not willing to properly educate ourselves on how to do it properly. When was the last time you saw an advertisement on television that preaches the importance, process, and exact steps needed in order to make exercise and eating properly a permanent part of your everyday hectic lifestyle? I've never seen one.

As you read through this entire book, you will see the logic and understand and master the process of weight loss and fitness whether you have 10 pounds or 100 pounds to shed.

Try to read the entire book, because in each chapter there are tidbits of information that are relevant no matter how much weight you need to lose. If you have a bad day or two, so be it, and continue on your quest for the *z*. As you persevere, you will make adjustments and corrections to your behavior and with time you will win. And remember to *only* think inside the box at all times and I promise you will be successful not only in meeting your weight-loss and fitness goals but also in every other aspect of your life!

Part I

EVERY DAY YOU THINK OUT-

SIDE THE BOX ADDS AN EXTRA

DAY OF NOT ACHIEVING YOUR

WEIGHT-LOSS AND FITNESS

GOALS!

CHAPTER ONE

What Does It Mean to Think Inside the Box?

Essentials

Every day, much like brushing your teeth, you need to pay attention to weight maintenance. In fact, most people will need to do so for their entire life in order to be successful in looking and performing their best. Look at it like any other chore: cutting your lawn, watering your plants, disciplining your child, working on your relationship, going to work, et cetera. When you focus on these issues and you put the time in and are consistent, it's safe to say you are happy with the outcome most of the time.

I have broken down all aspects in our life into what I call the Essentials. Your Essentials is your portfolio of life—all of the items represent what you *must* possess to have a happy, successful, and well-rounded life. There are four components that make up your Essentials: (1) **Lifestyle,** (2) **Career/Finances,** (3) **Fitness/Nutrition and Hobbies,** and (4) **Family Unit.**

Lifestyle	Career/Finances
Fitness/Nutrition and Hobbies	Family Unit

1. Your **Lifestyle** dictates how you live your everyday life: where you live, stress factors, how much you work, play, exercise, eat, and sleep, relaxation, the different types of pollution you're exposed to—in short, what your mind, body, and soul are exposed to on a day-in-and-day-out basis.

2. Your **Career/Finances** determine what kind of work you do, mental stimulation, how much you're learning and growing, sense of achievement both intrinsically and extrinsically, how much money you earn, the physical possessions you buy and gather, your financial stability, retirement funds, and how much leisure time you can carve out for yourself.

3. Your **Fitness/Nutrition and Hobbies** refer to your overall health, energy, fitness level, the type of foods you choose to eat, how you spend your idle time, time spent doing or performing non-work-related diversions, such as gardening, golf, tennis, hiking, fishing, reading, painting, stamp collecting, or anything else you enjoy doing.

4. Your **Family Unit** has to do with you, your partner, spouse, children, brothers, sisters, mother, father, cousins, aunts, grandparents, and any other relations, friends, and religious beliefs (if you have any).

Escape Route # 9: Life boils down to one word—*confidence!*

Although all four Essentials are necessary for sustaining life in some shape or form, the third Essential is the most important because it's the *catalyst* to ensuring that all the other three Essentials are being tended to.

How confident we are affects everything we attempt in our lifetime. The most effective way and, in my opinion, the *only* way you can sustain that confidence is by controlling how you feel about yourself. And let's face it: if you don't feel or look good or possess an energy or will to succeed, you cannot be on top of your game on a consistent basis. That's the true power of proper fitness—it is the most powerful, natural, mind- and body-altering drug known to mankind.

When you are attempting to lose weight and maintain weight loss, your main objective, as well as better health and more energy and productivity and looking your best, *can only* be achieved by organizing your daily activities to include proper fitness and good eating habits. So if you decide to not exercise or to try losing weight solely via a "new diet," you will fail.

Escape Route #10: Diets don't fail; people fail.

But the *reason* people fail is because they cannot sustain any diet that requires extremes, because no matter how much willpower you think you have, when the body is depleted or craves certain foods or nutrients and says "eat," you will eat and the pounds will come on even faster because of the additional calories you are now ingesting coupled with the fact that your BMR—the rate at which you burn and churn up calories during your resting state—has slowed to a snail's pace. This is just an example of how you are not thinking "inside the box," which I will be reminding you of each and every time you deviate from the blueprint of success that I am laying out for you.

It's not that difficult to lose some weight; the difficult part is keeping it off. And if you think back to when you initially lost some weight at one time or another and then gained it back, it was most likely due to the fact that you did not choose a plan that incorporated my last Escape Route. I purposely call these four components Essentials, because they are vital to our existence. Just as you put forward the effort to make more money or care for your grandparents or elderly parents, you must *pay attention* to Essential #3 in order to "have it all."

Escape Route #11: Before you choose to follow an exercise or eating plan you need to ask yourself whether you can follow this choice of path today, tomorrow, next week, next month, and for the rest of your life. If the answer is no, then you need to choose an alternate plan, specifically one that allows you to do all of the above.

Behaviors

That being said, over the last twenty years I have experienced three types of behavior that most people fall into who attempt to achieve weight loss and fitness: (1) those who "don't care" and are unwilling to change the fact that they are not exercising and are not willing to alter their eating habits, (2) those who "think" they're trying but are fooling themselves because they do it half-ass, and (3) those who are truly sincere and give 100 percent and are fanatics but unfortunately have either chosen the wrong plan or chosen a course of action that is missing some key ingredients.

Some individuals actually have exhibited all three of these behaviors at different times in their lives to achieve weight loss and fitness. Some people live in denial and only experience one of these behaviors in their quest to look and feel their best. As you'll soon learn by reading part 1 of this book, it's not enough and by no means a guarantee that just because you're trying that you'll be successful *unless* the plan and path you choose make sense on a day-in-and-day-out basis.

I'd like to make something very clear to all of you reading this book. I don't care what I need to do to change your behavior and make you re-think your weight-loss and fitness goals. As long as it's honest, moral, and ethical, I will use any means necessary to help you feel and look your best. I am and will be sensitive to you when I need to be. But I cannot allow you to manipulate me and control the situation. Besides, what do you do for a living again? Oh, that's right, you are an investment banker, and because of your years of experience in the motivational and fitness industry I'm supposed to listen to you in regard to weight loss and fitness. Just as your clients, because they go to the bank and deposit money, feel confident guiding you and telling you which investment opportunities you should consider and which you should steer clear from. It's called *tough love*. I am very proud of the fact that I have over an 80 percent success rate with my clients. Considering that the national percentage for weight loss is about 2 or 3 percent, I'd say that mine is pretty darn good, and I know that if my stockbroker were as successful as I am, I would be writing this book from a castle rather than my NYC apartment.

That killer, tenacious, and passionate attitude that I exude is what I am trying to give you, the reader. You need to attack your weight-loss and fitness regimen with energy and the attitude that no matter what curveball life throws at you, you will overcome all of them and succeed!

The following narratives are true-life experiences that I want to share with you in order to make certain points or emphasize a particular position. Identify with one or more of these behaviors and apply the resolution to the problem to get your mind-set to thinking inside the box.

Behavior Type #1—*Laissez-Faire*

Dilemma: You "don't really care" how you look and how you are perceived by others. Now, take a step back and think about this. I put "don't really care" in quotes because of course you "care" about how you look and feel and what you exude and don't exude to others around you. What it really boils down to is that it is not a *priority* or important enough for you to change for the better. And it doesn't matter the true reason or why you don't care. You could just be plain lazy or loathe exercise, you have tried many attempts to lose weight but have failed in the past, you work long hours and are too tired to exercise, your hectic lifestyle prevents you from incorporating a sound eating and fitness plan into your daily activities, or perhaps you have a physical or orthopedic condition and use that as your reasoning for not achieving weight loss and fitness. Whatever the excuse, constraint, or reasoning, it just isn't important enough for you to regroup, rethink, and make any or another futile attempt to lose weight and become fit. But funny enough, you have plenty of time and make the following examples a priority in your life. Here are a few stories that I have personally experienced and have witnessed over the years:

The building in which our Exude Fitness facility is located in midtown Manhattan also happens to have a day spa. We are on the third floor, and the spa is on the second floor. I can't tell you how many *hundreds* of times I have stepped on the elevator and it was about to close when I heard "hold the elevator." Rushing in with vim and vigor are these women and men who run in and hit the second-floor button. As I look at these people

Escape Route #12:
When was the last time you were honest with yourself, gave 100 percent, and failed at that endeavor? I bet it is far less than the number of times you failed because of a lack of effort.

I can't but notice how nicely put together they appear—perfectly dyed hair, impeccably dressed with all the gold jewelry, et cetera, et cetera—they are also yet vastly overweight and unhealthy-looking. So I chuckle and say to myself, *You'll run to get your nails manicured, hair dyed, and yourself pampered, but you won't run to get in shape? You make your hair and nails a priority but not your body? Trust me, honey, I ain't looking at your nails; besides, I cannot get past how you ignore your body. You'll spend hundreds of dollars and two hours to dye your hair, but you can't find it in yourself to spend four hours a week to get your butt in shape.* Besides, that short-lived feeling about how "good" you think you look gets all washed away the next morning after you shower. And you guys out there will spend thousands of dollars on a new car, worrying about every little nick and scratch and how cool you think you look in that sports convertible, but God forbid you spend a dollar on getting rid of your gut.

How about the fine restaurants people eat in every day? You'll also spend a few hundred dollars on a fine dinner to stuff yourself or thousands on a new couch to sit on your duff but refuse to spend any money on a stationary bike or treadmill that will actually *allow* you to enjoy that meal or new couch even more and without guilt!

There is an upside to every vastly overweight person out there. It takes an enormous amount of money to get that big in the first place. You didn't become 50 pounds or more overweight by not eating—a lot and often—and eating or drinking that much requires spending money. A monthly health club membership is certainly within reach of your budget, but only if you want to start eating less and applying those savings toward bettering yourself. This requires educating yourself on how to start a fitness regimen within your budget, but not before you make it a *priority*, just as you have made eating a priority.

Solutions: There are a number of ways to help you make proper fitness and better eating habits a priority in your life. For instance, sometimes how you view yourself may not be how others view you. Ask your partner, spouse, or friend to take a picture of you in underwear for guys and a bra and underpants for women. Take that picture and put it on your mirror. Now ask yourself this question. What turns you off more, the thought of having to exercise and eat sensibly or how you feel when you look at your picture? If you are happy with the way you look, then fine, accept yourself as you are, but don't complain about how you look and feel. If life is great, you are happy with your body, your self-esteem is great, and you don't feel a need for change, keep eating. But if you don't like how you look in that picture, make a promise to yourself that you are going to start a fitness program and develop better eating habits so

Escape Route #13: We tend to take better care of our automotive vehicles than the vehicles in which we drive around in 24 hours a day—our bodies!

that you can start in making proper fitness a consistent part of your life. Depending upon your weight-loss goals, select the plan most applicable to you and start moving!

You can also choose a hobby, sport, or activity that you might enjoy doing on a regular basis, such as basketball, skiing, tennis, golf, gardening, et cetera. If you have a child or children, spend more time with them doing these things. It takes a certain fitness level to keep up with children and if you want to spend more time with them, you're going to need to get in shape. Besides, if you want your children to grow up and be fit, it is necessary to start them off at an early age. Or perhaps you want to start gardening, which by the way is a wonderful form of exercise but can be very demanding. Getting in better shape will allow you to garden more effectively and longer and, most important, allow you to enjoy it more because you won't be huffing and puffing each time you bend over to plant, pick weeds, or grade your garden. Whatever activity you choose, it is a wonderful motivator because your focus can be directed toward becoming more efficient at your hobby; thus you will enjoy it more rather than focusing solely on a regimented fitness plan. And for some, especially those who don't enjoy formal exercise or loathe it, it can be the difference between remaining out of shape for the rest of their lives and not.

Escape Route #14: It doesn't matter what means you use to motivate yourself to exercise or why you choose to do so; as long as it gets you moving, it's effective!

Behavior Type #2—*Dreamer*

Dilemma: You work out a few days a week and eat decently, yet you don't really see enough progress and are always complaining that "it isn't working." You are not willing to change your mode (type) of exercise and cannot understand that with all your efforts you're not Miss or Mr. America yet.

I call this type of people dreamers because you're dreaming if you think that just because you are "exercising" you are entitled to pass Go and collect $200.00. You're kidding yourself because you are still unwilling to truly work hard and make small adjustments to your everyday eating and drinking habits. Sure, you go to the gym two or three days per week, but you are either not exercising properly or not exercising intensely enough (you only walk on a treadmill). Or you need to shed weight and you partake in passive exercise but ignore the fact that aerobic activity is what you need to be doing in order to shed that excess weight. Yoga, Pilates, and other forms of exercise, combined with aerobic exercise, would do the trick, but you don't "like" to do certain exercises and are not capable of opening your eyes to see the whole field. You'll spend some money on a health club or classes but are not willing to spend money on hiring a personal trainer because you cannot see the value in doing so. I call you a

Burger King child, not because you eat fast food but because you want to do it "your way," not the right way. You are also the type that comes into my facility with more diamonds and gold than Pharaoh himself but balks when I hand you a price list and responds, "It's so expensive; I can't afford it." And I have no problem whatsoever countering with, "You can afford it; you choose not to afford it. Sell one of your antiques or one of your five gold chains dangling from your neck, and then you can afford it. You're going to spend the money anyway, so you might as well get back something positive. Instead of going shopping to find the dress or suit that doesn't make you look so big, save your money and put some dough toward making your body look good so that you feel and look great in anything you possess in your closet."

Another common saga of the dreamer tells how when I lay out an exact fitness plan he/she meets with our nutritionist and then proceeds to do exactly the opposite of what he/she just paid us for.

"Edward, I didn't learn anything from the nutritionist."

"Oh, really?" I respond. "It's funny, looking at her notes on you, you eat out seven days per week, ordering appetizers, a main course, three drinks, and then dessert. I'm sure that Hillary [one of our nutritionists] ignored these facts and gave you carte blanche to eat whatever and whenever you desire and to *not* alter your eating habits. And thirty days later when you complain to my staff that 'it isn't working,' I then sit you down and review the guarantee I sent you when you came on board as a client. It specifically says and you agreed that you would follow the plan that we outlined for fitness and nutrition. In addition, you were supposed to make small dietary changes, of which you have made none, and do your fitness homework two or three days per week specifically outlined with aerobic activity for thirty minutes, stretches, and abdominal exercises to help your tummy area. Again, you *choose* not to do it. Now you can easily see why 'you're not working.' Your sense of entitlement is mind-boggling. You are still making the same mistakes you made with your weight-loss and fitness goals *prior* to coming in here. You are dreaming if you think you will ever change the way you look and feel unless you stop fighting yourself, me, and the system and are willing to yield and listen. And I don't care if you don't 'like' it. There's no rule in life that we must 'like' everything in our lives that is good for us. Hey, if you have to pick up your child after school on a day when you are exhausted, it's raining, and there's tons of traffic, do you not go and pick up your child because 'you don't like it'? Of course not. You suck it up and act responsibly.

"Well, guess what? You need to be responsible to yourself as well. And I don't care if it's fitness, love, work, family, or whatever—you need to rechannel all of that energy and change your mind-set. Stop searching for a shortcut and start realizing that in order to become more attractive to yourself and others you need to be honest with yourself and try a different game plan, because the one you are now following is not working! In short, you have a "bad" relationship with your fitness and lifestyle program. You can either "stay" in this relationship or reach down and have the strength and drop it like a bomb. But if you decide to stay in this predicament, know the shortcomings and accept them. If you truly want to better how you look and feel, you need to clear your mind and start over again with a "new" relationship *without* bringing your dirty laundry to the table. Dreamers have the hardest time adapting and adjusting to a new fitness and diet plan because they like to call the shots and are not used to being told what to do. Learn to give up just a bit of control and to yield and you'll be successful in reaching your weight-loss goals.

Solutions: Start by slowly breaking away from what you do normally with exercise and diet. Do not go to extremes. In other words, if you typically dine out most of the week, don't think of or try only dining out once or twice a week. (1) You'll be miserable, and (2) you'll never adhere to it. Instead, you should educate yourself on how to eat out sensibly by learning how to more wisely spend your calories through eating and drinking.

Instead of a fattening appetizer, choose a salad. Split a full portion with your partner, or if you are dining alone, order a half-portion. If you drink, order wine spritzers; then you can drink four of them but are only consuming the alcohol and caloric content of two glasses of wine and will still be satisfied. Cut down your desserts to either two days per week and use them as a reward for working out hard that particular day. If you do just the above, in one week you will have consumed nearly half the calories you typically do and will lose weight in no time *without* having to have "given" up anything.

For your exercise, if you are so adamant about taking a particular class a few days a week (remember, it isn't working, although it does make you feel good), do 30 minutes of aerobic exercise before or after the class or take it only once a week so that you don't have withdrawal symptoms, and do your formal exercise program the other days based upon your weight-loss goals (see chapter 5, 6, 7 and 8).

Another effective way of reaching your fitness and weight-loss goals is to set up a reward system for yourself. The reward can be intrinsic or extrinsic in nature; it doesn't matter. Like receiving a massage: I'm always fascinated by the number of massages that people who are completely unfit get. In my opinion, they haven't deserved the massages. But if you work out hard and eat properly, suddenly that massage will feel a lot better because it kind of validates what and why you have been working at so hard to achieve. In other words, you've *earned* it.

Behavior Type #3—*Extremist*

Dilemma: I once went out to dinner with a group of friends and a couple of clients. As we all settled down and started to order our dishes, I reached for some bread and then proceeded to actually put butter on that piece of bread. All of a sudden, I heard out of nowhere: "I can't believe you eat butter, Edward, especially because of the industry you're in."

Totally taken aback, I responded, "I can't believe you *don't* eat butter and look the way you do." Aside from the fact that she was at least 30 pounds overweight, she was so obsessed about every little thing she and others were putting in their mouths, she didn't have a clue as to how to eat properly and also enjoy her life. Let me tell you something: if I can't go out for dinner and eat an occasional piece of bread (with butter on it of course) and enjoy a drink or two, then you know what? Life is not worth living. That's one of the reasons that I exercise and exercise properly, so that I can indulge from time to time and eat whatever I desire, as long as I do it in moderation. Remember, it doesn't matter what motivates you to exercise properly and regularly; that doesn't change or alter the benefits.

You've seen them and you know the type. They either follow a strict vegetarian diet or go on a no-carbohydrate diet or exercise seven days per week for two hours each stint and gorge themselves just as often. They are so stressed out worrying what they're putting in their system that the stress alone is doing more harm than good and it is this stress and worry that is actually "killing" them.

They are nonconforming and resistant to change. They go away to these ashrams and follow the tutelage of some wacko who tries to sell you their "spiritual" tapes, and it is borderline cultish. You'll enjoy this story. About ten years ago I received a phone call from one of Guru Myra's disciples in an ashram in upstate New York. The disciple asked me if I could see some of their top counselors to design fitness programs for them at what was then my very small exercise studio. I decided to see them in groups, two or three at a time. Shockingly, I wasn't prepared for what I was about to experience. Everyone from this ashram who came to me (the counselors) was in such poor physical condition that I could have taken a stranger off the street and he/she would have been more fit, and yet these counselors were teaching yoga and other fitness-related courses where you, the consumer, pays hundreds of dollars. In addition to being unfit, nearly 80 percent of the counselors had one or more eating disorders, terrible teeth, and suffered from borderline depression.

> *Escape Route #17:*
> Weight loss, eating, and drinking are all about checks and balances, specifically calories in versus calories out. And those who can best balance their checkbooks are never in over their heads.

They also had another common denominator: most of them were run-aways. Having traveled across the country, these once homeless and desperate individuals thought that they had found their safe haven at the ashram. So I say to myself, as any other rational person would, how can any of these counselors possibly guide me to the road of better fitness if they themselves aren't fit? After a month or so of helping the counselors, I was asked to go up to the ashram and give a lecture to all of them. The wealth up there was astonishing. The auditorium I spoke in could easily have rivaled Carnegie Hall, with its gold-laden drapes, velvet chairs, and huge seating capacity. Next up, I am to meet Guru Mayra herself.

She was quite beautiful, with an entourage of bodyguards, and was completely surrounded by dozens of small children who appeared almost under her spell. As we were introduced to each other, she extended her hand to mine, and as I went to shake her hand, an electric bolt from my hand shot out when our hands met, and she quickly turned away and realized that the jig was up. I had her number, and she knew she couldn't manipulate me into buying into the ashram's ruse. Hey, at least they paid their bill to me. So, the next time you want to "better" your life, do your research before you spend your hard-earned money and time, whether it's on spas, health clubs, massage, et cetera.

Another extremist behavior I have witnessed over the years involves the guys and gals out there with the runner's mentality. All they do is run, perhaps up to ten miles daily; meanwhile their bodies look a tad undernourished, with poor flexibility, no muscle tone, and weak upper body strength, and they have more orthopedic problems than a racing car crash victim and will not under any circumstances exercise any other way. These are the same type of people who come into my facility with a certain mind-set and ask for help yet fight me or challenge everything I say because it is contraindicative of what their "trainer" has told them or "what I've read." If I had a dollar for every time I heard "that's not what my trainer told me," I'd be retired today. So, I counter with, "If your trainer knew what was right for you, (a) you wouldn't be here, and (b) you would be fit, and (c) I would be working for this trainer and he/she, not I, would own the largest and most successful motivational and fitness company in the country." That being said, I explain that a lot of trainers out there are very good at teaching you proper form and technique, and are truly sincere in helping you get in better shape. But there is a huge difference between teaching someone how to perform exercises with proper form *and* designing a proper fitness and eating plan that takes into consideration that person's goals, lifestyle, medical and orthopedic background, and current level of fitness. They are like apples and oranges; both are pieces of fruit but vastly different. For instance, at Exude unless you are a registered dietician and licensed in the state of New York, you are not allowed to give *any* advice as to diet, supplements, vitamins, et cetera. And it is no accident that after being in business for nearly 20 years we have never even had a liability claim or lawsuit against our company. That is not luck. It is due to the fact that we only allow true experts to give advice to our clients, not some uneducated, inexperienced mirror-loving lad who only knows how to lift a weight. And remember, just because someone is an expert in his/her field doesn't guarantee that he/she is equally impactful in teaching it.

I personally have seen and worked with over 20,000 individuals over the years and during this time I can honestly say that I have never had an extremist type walk into my facility who was truly fit. Sure they were "fit" to run or fit in some arenas, but overall fitness—no. I have also worked with thousands of thin "fatties." These people in clothes look slender, trim, and somewhat fit. But when they are in gym clothes you can see they are clinically obese, meaning that 30 percent or more of their total body weight is fat. Vegetarians and those who follow fat-free diets are more likely to fall into this category. The misconception is that if we only eat certain foods or avoid certain food groups it will make us look and feel great.

Nine out of ten women I have seen over the years have cellulite in some region of their body, and in some cases, the thinner they are, the more cellulite they possess. American and Asian women, that is. Europeans, South Americans, African-Americans, and women from Third World nations tend to have far less cellulite. I know it's because of their diets. Americans and Asians tend to eat more carbohydrates and high-starch-type foods, whereas the other groups eat a diet richer in fats and oils, which seems to lubricate their skin and allow it to be more elastic.

As you read on and explore the chapters coming up on nutrition and dietary plans, I employed the services of Hillary Baron, R.D., to help me design the proper eating plans and guidelines because I needed her expertise to give me accurate information so that I could organize it in a way that is safe and effective for you, the reader.

Solutions: Extremists need to take a step back and open their minds to change, learn to relax, not worry about every little thing, especially those things over which they have no control. They also need to stop listening to every so-called guru out there and ask themselves before they try a particular route to weight loss and fitness if the plan they are considering can be followed *without* denying themselves anything. Also, they need to restructure their fitness regimen and make it more complete, one that incorporates all five components of fitness: cardiovascular conditioning,

Escape Route #18: Your diet or food intake affects more your scale weight, not necessarily your shape or muscle tone. Only proper exercise can make your body look and be fit as well as raise your BMR.

muscle endurance, muscle strength, flexibility, and body ratio, ensuring they possess a fit and toned body throughout. I always describe extremists this way: they study chapters 1–5, but the final exam covers chapters 1–10. These people are perfect examples of receiving an A for effort and an F for completion.

Another effective way of breaking the extremist mentality is to align yourself with people who are not as obsessed with weight loss and fitness as yourself. A key suggestion is to focus and channel your energy to improving yourself by making your regimens more well rounded rather than focusing solely on the outcome. It's like golfers who are so focused and concerned with shooting a particular score rather than just going out there and enjoying themselves and focusing on the task one hole at a time. If you have a bad hole, put it behind you and don't let it carry over to the next hole or holes; otherwise you will stress yourself out over things that haven't even happened yet. If you are adamant about eating or exercising a certain way, try to take a day or two and push yourself to try an alternate plan. See how you feel after a few weeks, and before you know it you will slowly be better at accepting change for the better. Most important, look in the mirror and honestly ask yourself if what you see you love. Ask a close friend or your partner what he/she thinks about your "look." Often we are too close and too emotionally attached to give an unbiased opinion of ourselves. And that's okay. What's not okay is not being open-minded enough to make the necessary adjustments to continually improve ourselves.

I've put together a balance sheet of sorts that will help you in achieving weight loss and improving your fitness level. As you are now realizing, weight loss and fitness is not just about eating properly and working out. A number of other components "add" to the pie. I call this balance sheet a **Habit Atlas** because it tracks your weekly activity, fitness, and eating habits. There is a scoring system based on these three factors and a rating scale on your particular habits that will help guide you in meeting your weight-loss and fitness goals. Your grading system is on a weekly basis.

All you need to do is take a snapshot of your week based on this grading system and you'll easily see why you are losing weight, maintaining your current weight, or gaining weight. It's all about calories in versus calories out. And as you can see, there are a few ways that you can reach your weight-loss and fitness goals. However, you cannot get there *by* only choosing or mastering one habit.

Escape Route #19:
Weight loss and fitness is not just about working hard; it's about working effectively.

Escape Route #20:
Weight loss, weight management, and fitness is something we need to pay attention to for our entire lives, not just for a month or on a part-time basis, and when we can accept this fact *only* then can we meet most of our goals and objectives.

Your Habit Atlas is your road map, sort of your blueprint to follow in order to achieve all of your weight-loss and fitness goals. So even if you have the discipline to eat well seven days a week while not exercising or exercise six days a week while not eating well, you still would not score that high. You should strive for two activities per week, five workouts per week, and five good-eating days, which will give you a total score of 27 points. Your lifestyle will dictate your activity days and some of your fitness days. Poor preparation based upon your lifestyle will dictate your good eating days, not your lifestyle by itself. Based on this atlas, if you have to "cheat," cheat with the lower scoring habits of activities and/or good eating days because you can make it up with your fitness days. You cannot, however, make up for so few exercise days no matter how well you eat or active you are. Your goal is to try to duplicate a good or better score week in and week out.

You should strive for three out of four weeks to score well so that if you have a bad week every month or so, you are still way ahead of the game and will eventually win at weight loss and fitness. This is the best example of what I mean by thinking inside the box.

I MUST BE OPEN TO CHANGE,

BECAUSE USING MY CURRENT

WAY OF THINKING AND WHAT I

THINK I KNOW ABOUT

EXERCISE AND FITNESS

OBVIOUSLY IS NOT WORKING.

CHAPTER TWO

Facts Versus Fallacies on Exercise and Fitness

We have heard, read, and been told many misconceptions concerning exercise in general and what to avoid, and this could mean the difference between success and failure in our search for weight loss. So I've put together a number of these fitness faux pas to save you time and, more important, help you avoid these traps *before* you even *think* of buying into any of them. Although there are hundreds of these, I've put together the top 15 in a quiz format of fact versus myth. It's also important for you, the reader, to feel comfortable that *all* of the information regarding these facts versus myths is medically proven. It's not the world according to Edward Jackowski; it's data unknown to the layperson, whose purpose is to alert and educate you with accurate information. What you do with this information is up to you. I hope you will heed my advice and make these adjustments into your own personal fitness regimen or, if you don't have one as of yet, take stock and be aware of them. See if you know the facts versus the myths and grade yourself at the end.

Fact or Myth #1: **Muscle weighs more than fat.** On your kitchen table you have five pounds of fat, five pounds of muscle, five pounds of gold, five pounds of potatoes, and five pounds of feathers. Which weighs more? Actually, they *all* weigh the same; five pounds is five pounds. What people mean to say is that per square inch of volume or space the weight of muscle is more dense than that of fat. Imagine making a fist. That is about the space that one pound of fat takes up. Now take your thumb and forefinger and make a circle with your fingers; this silver dollar of space represents the space or volume that one pound of muscle takes up. Pound for pound, fat takes up approximately 2.5 times the amount of space as muscle. Because fat takes up more space, that's one of the reasons people who possess a lot of fat actually look and appear *heavier* than they are and people with a healthier body fat ratio look *lighter* than the scale indicates or to the naked eye. Now, can't we fit or insert a lot more of those silver dollars versus fists in our body?

Answer: **Myth.**

Fact or Myth #2: **Lifting moderate to heavy weights is the most effective way of creating a healthier body ratio which will allow me to burn more fat and help me to lose weight.** This is perhaps the most popular misconception circulating out there today. What do cross-country skiers, swimmers, marathon runners, ballet dancers, and triathletes have in common? That's right: none of these athletes are heavy or possess a lot of mass. Based on the theory that one *needs* to lift weights in order to burn fat more efficiently, then all of these athletes should be heavy, because they lift little or no weights in their exercise regimens. Moreover, how come athletes in the early 1900s and before that time who participated in any of these types of sports were built similar to today's athletes who partake in these same sports or activities? Belief in this faux pas is doing a grave injustice today by causing all the millions of women out there—who think that if they lift weights their metabolism will work more efficiently and that they will be able to burn more fat because they will possess more muscle.

In *theory,* this is true. But what you, the layperson, and, for that matter, even professionals in the fitness industry don't know is that in order to raise your Basal Metabolic Rate through weight lifting—known as your BMR—the human body needs to put on approximately 20 percent more muscle mass in order to raise its BMR by just 5 percent. Considering that most people are overweight today, they are not in a position to **add** mass to their body. And just because you are lifting weights and getting stronger doesn't guarantee that your BMR is going to be more efficient, because you could be lifting weights with low to moderate repetitions (reps) or lifting a heavy weight that requires lots of rest in between each set or exercise, thus not working intensely enough in order to effectively raise your BMR.

In fact, based on the theory that we *need* to lift weights in order to have a healthier body fat ratio, then every single human walking around the face of this earth (including myself) who does not lift weights *should* be fat and have an inefficient BMR. Are you beginning to see my point? So, I still haven't told you why the athletes that I mentioned earlier are not fat and obviously possess an efficient BMR. They own an efficient fat-burning body primarily because when they do work out and exercise they work out with enough intensity to allow them to burn fat during exercise for hours afterward. It is the *intensity* at which we exercise that allows us to possess a healthier body fat ratio, which then allows us to burn more calories during our resting state, and **not** the *type* of exercise per se. In addition, weights and resistance come in many forms. For instance, a typical female ballet dancer may weigh about 120 pounds. Each and every time she lifts her legs or body repetitively, she is moving 120 pounds! Now just because there isn't a weight or dumbbell attached to her body doesn't mean she is not lifting enough weight. Actually her body is so lithe because she *only* lifts her body as her sole weight and resistance. If she added more weights to her routine she would possess more mass and (1) it would look awkward and (2) she would not be able to move with the ease and grace that we admire and respect when we watch ballet dancers.

Answer: **Myth.**

Fact or Myth #3: **Walking is one of best exercises anyone can do for weight loss and to combat osteoporosis.** Hey, if all we needed to do to look great and possess a fit and toned body was walk, then why are most people overweight and unfit? Especially if you live in a major city or any other environment where you walk all the time, one would think that is enough to trim us or give us any number of fitness or health-related benefits. I am not saying that walking is bad for you, nor am I saying that it cannot be *part* of a fitness regimen. But by itself, walking does not represent fitness. Why? Because fitness as defined in medical terms, not *your* interpretation, is comprised of five elements or components: flexibility, cardiovascular conditioning, muscle strength, muscle endurance, and body ratio. What this means to you, the layperson, is that if we want to *improve* or increase our fitness levels, *each and every time* we choose to exercise we must exercise in a fashion that addresses or hits all five components. Now that you know this, it's easy to see why walking by *itself* is not fitness but rather an example of an exercise.

Don't fret, because there is no one exercise in and of itself that does represent total fitness. And that includes jogging, running, aerobic, step, or any other exercise classes, Pilates, yoga, weight lifting, Spinning, kickboxing, et cetera. And just because you do choose to walk as a form of exercise, you still need to warm up, stretch, walk intensely, and then cool down to even allow your body to improve cardiovascularly.

Another misconception is that walking is great for combating osteoporosis. Well, again that depends on how long you walk, the intensity at which you walk, and how frequently you walk. Walking does virtually

Escape Route #21: Although "fitness" is plausibly simple, it actually is a lot more complex than people realize and there is a lot more to it than meets the eye.

Escape Route #22: If you are exercising a certain way for 30 days or more and your body is not changing for the better in the areas you want it to, stop, because you're exercising wrong!

Escape Route #23:
When trying to lose mass, the heavier you are, the lighter weights you need to use, and conversely, when trying to add mass, the lighter you are, the heavier the weights you should use to give your body a more balanced and symmetrical appearance. So, if you want to trim down, don't despair, because now you know that all you have to do is use light weights with more repetitions combined with performing more aerobic-type exercise to reach your goals!

little or nothing to alter your bone density for your upper body because it isn't weight-bearing for your upper body. So if you do suffer from or are susceptible to osteoporosis from the waist up, you still need to perform weight-bearing exercises that address and attack the regions of your upper body where your bone density needs to be increased.

Answer: **Myth.**

Fact or Myth #4: **Squats, lunges, and leg presses are excellent ways to trim the buttocks, legs, and hips.** This one is my favorite. I cannot tell you how many women out there today are bulking up, adding mass, and doing the exact opposite of what they are seeking to do: trimming and eliminating fat and mass from their lower extremities.

What's more unbelievable is that these same women are squatting and lunging away because "my trainer says that if I lift more weights I will possess more muscle and thus burn more fat." Well, now that you are more educated and know the facts surrounding this faux pas, what are you going to do about it? It's uncanny and one of the few things I have not mastered yet that for the life of me I cannot comprehend how intelligent people ignore the fact that their body is not trimming down and *for years* keep exercising the same way, hoping, praying, that someday, as if by magic, their body will suddenly take a turn for the better and it will start to shrink rather than bulk up. Here's the skinny on this matter: the heavier you are, the faster you will bulk up when you apply moderate to heavy weights or resistance during exercise. To further prove my point, are weight lifters skinny or bulky? So when you hear or read something that says women who lift weights *won't* bulk up, ask yourself this question: How come professional bodybuilders, men and women alike, don't swim or jog for their mode of exercise? Based on that theory that weights don't bulk, then you or I could garden or play badminton and possess the same body mass and compete with bodybuilders in their next competition, because remember, weights don't bulk. Think about this: take a photo of a marathon runner and a picture of a bodybuilder and switch their workouts—the marathon runner only lifts weights for one year and the body builder runs 10 miles a day for the year. After the year, take another picture of both. Now you're going to tell me that they will still possess the same body after a year of altering their workouts?

Get it yet? Of course weights bulk. And some people who are either bottom- or top-heavy or both will bulk up even faster while using even moderate weights. Everyone has a formula that they need to adhere to when trying to lose weight rather than tone muscles.

Answer: **Myth.**

Fact or Myth #5: **To firm the fat on the back of your arms, triceps, kick-backs, push-ups, and push-downs are all effective exercises.** If this were true, then every gal and guy who performed any or all of these exercises should have perfect arms. In my twenty years of meeting many thousands of women of all ages, I would have to say that only one out of a thousand have perfect arms, perfect in the sense of size, symmetry, tone, and how they look compared to the rest of the body. The factual and medical reason that none of the above exercises or movements will firm the fat on the back of your arms is that *fat* and *muscle* are composed of different substances. Fat *cannot* be converted to muscle and muscle *does not* turn to fat.

So, the next time you want to tone your flabby arms, take a step back before you start lifting with a simple kick-back with dumbbells, and be aware that no exercise can firm the flab on the back of your arms. Oh, I forgot to tell you something equally significant: this doesn't just apply to the fat on the back of your arms but fat throughout your body as well—including the fat on your inner and outer thigh region, hips, stomach, calves, back, chest, and wherever on your body you need to "firm up."

Now that you know that it is not possible to firm the fat on the back of your arms or in any other region of your body, what are you to do? Although it's true that when you lift that dumbbell during your kick-backs you will burn calories and fat, for some the rate at which you are building muscle is *faster* than the rate at which you are burning fat, especially if you are overweight or genetically you hold more fat in that particular region of your body. When we tax or work our muscles with moderate to high weight/resistance, the muscle responds by growing. That's why bodybuilders and athletes who exercise using a lot of weights/resistance in their exercise regimens get "pumped up." Combining excess fat you have in a particular section of your body with this lifting results in an increase of girth to that region of your body being worked.

Remember the examples I gave earlier in Myth #4 of the marathon runner and why he/she is slender and weight lifters are bulky? The reason their bodies look this way is the *type* of exercise they perform. Aerobic exercise, such as running, walking, jogging, swimming, jumping rope, et cetera, in addition to improving cardiovasculaar efficiency helps take mass/weight off the body, and anaerobic-type exercises such as sit-ups, weight lifting, push-ups, et cetera, are best suited for toning or building muscles. So, if you're overweight and want to trim your arms or any other part of your body as well as tone up in that particular region of your body, you need to perform lots of low-resistance aerobic exercise

Escape Route #24: There exists no exercise or exercises that can firm fat in any area of the human body.

combined with some anaerobic (toning) exercises using *extremely* low weights and high repetitions.

Answer: **Myth.**

Fact or Myth #6: **Yoga, Pilates, The Firm, cardio kickboxing, and other popular fad-type exercise classes are excellent fitness regimens.** Although these forms of exercise can offer health/fitness benefits by themselves, they do not represent true "fitness." The major reason why, aside from the fact that no one exercise in and of itself represents proper fitness (see Myth #3), is that it is extremely difficult to find the intensity level at which one needs to be exercising while performing these exercise routines in a class setting. The instructor performs a move while you, the class participant, perform the same move, but it is nearly impossible for that instructor to be exercising while ensuring that everyone in classs is properly aligned, using correct form, and exercising at a safe and effective target heart rate zone. In addition, what may be intense enough for one participant may be too much or not nearly intense enough for an extremely fit individual to reap enough fitness benefits.

That is just one of a thousand logical reasons I can give you why *very few* people are able to reach their fitness and weight-loss goals in a large-class format. One of my "hobbies" I enjoy while traveling is visiting at least one type of gym or health club or spa on each trip. I do so for a number of reasons: (1) to see what new trends are popping up, (2) to observe class participants and watch people in general as to how they are exercising, and (3) to watch people's efforts while they are working out. And I have to tell you, whether it's New York, Texas, California, Europe, the Caribbean, or Canada, no one has a clue as to what they are doing when it comes to performing a complete fitness regimen, one that encompasses all five components of fitness with the frequency, duration, and intensity that will even allow more than subtle changes. I can walk through a gym or glance in at any exercise class going on in any part of the world and see the same mistakes being made over and over and I just cringe, because I know that nearly 90 percent of these people will never ever reach any of their weight-loss *or* fitness goals. From people not keeping up with the instructor to individuals performing the exercise with improper form, compromising their health because they are stressing their joints or arching their back or jerking the weight as they are lowering it toward their body, it goes on and on. Here's my favorite: people come to class early and reserve the same step or position in class by waiting outside the classroom, sometimes for up to 30 minutes, sitting on their duff doing nothing. Of course, most of these people are the same guys and gals who are vastly overweight and out-of-shape. Hey, did you ever think of spending that 20 minutes or more sitting on your ass riding a recumbent exercise bike so that you can reap some fitness benefits? Of course not. It's as if these people are so programmed that they cannot move a muscle until the instructor shows up. God forbid he/she is late or doesn't show up for a class; then what would they do, keep waiting until the next day? Don't get me wrong, I think exercise classes are an excellent way of providing motivation and support to many exercisers out there, but you should never allow yourself to be put in the position of complete dependency upon them or you will never learn to properly exercise on your own. Besides, that class is not the answer-all to your fitness and weight-loss needs; it's incomplete by itself anyway.

Answer: **Myth.**

Fact or Myth #7: **It's important to stretch** *before* **and** *after* **each time you work out.** Yes, it is important to stretch each and every time you work out, but *when* you stretch is equally important. Stretching should only take place *after* you have warmed up. The reason: warming up raises your core body temperature, which allows you to improve blood circulation to your muscles, which will improve the elasticity to your joints and muscles. In addition, warming up *prior* to stretching allows the area being stretched to better align with your joints, thus creating better posture, balance, and symmetry throughout your entire body. I always hear "Did you warm up?" "Yeah, I stretched already." Or "Did you stretch?" "Yeah, I warmed up." The two are not synonymous and should not be interpreted or substituted for each other. They are two distinct and different phases of fitness.

> *Escape Route #25:* Don't rely solely on the "buddy" system for exercise or fitness, because when your "buddy" doesn't show up, you won't, either.

There are four phases to fitness: warm-up, stretch, workload, and cooldown. And according to the American College of Sports Medicine (ACSM), each time we engage in an exercise routine we must follow this protocol in this exact order so that our bodies can absorb the benefits of fitness, in addition to lowering our risk of injury and, yes, death! You would be shocked how many people cannot even name the four phases of a workout or the five components that make up a proper fitness regimen. So, if you don't even know these ever-so-important facts, how can you possibly imagine or dream that your body will ever change? It can't, and that's why certain people who are "exercising" are not able to reach any of their weight-loss or fitness goals, but do injure themselves and put undue stress on their joints. And trainers are the worst culprits of all. I can't tell you how many of our past and existing clientele at Exude never warmed up or stretched prior to performing their core workout routine despite the fact that they all had worked with a trainer in the past. They look at me completely bewildered, as if I am speaking Russian to them.

By the way, every nationally certified trainer in this country takes an exam and has been educated on the importance of warming up and stretching *prior* to working out, but because they are "Burger Kings" they want to do it "their way" and not the correct way, many of these people don't even warm up and stretch themselves. One of the main reasons that most people don't warm up, then stretch before they exercise is because they don't know the proper techniques or what's involved in doing so. They know that they should be doing something along the lines of this but don't possess the knowledge to do it; thus they blow it off.

Escape Route #26: There is a direct correlation between education and motivation when it comes to exercise and fitness; the more you know, the more apt you are to do what's needed.

One of the misconceptions about stretching is that it prevents injury. In essence, this is somewhat correct, but it is not infallible. However, warming up and stretching properly definitely helps prevent serious injury. For instance, if you have stretched and you perform a movement or exercise that doesn't agree with your body, that stretching could mean the difference between straining your muscle and pulling or tearing your muscle. And by increasing your flexibility you also increase your range of motion, which benefits you because you put less stress on your joints as well as increase the amount of calories you are burning while exercising. Stretching *after* your workout will increase your flexibility as well, but you still need to stretch *before* you work out. Be careful, though, when you do stretch after your workout that you don't overstretch any muscle group that you just heavily worked or taxed, because by overstretching you increase your chances of straining or pulling those particular muscles that you just exercised.

Answer: **Myth.**

Fact or Myth #8: **We burn more calories and fat during long sustained aerobic activity, which is why we need to perform at least 20 minutes of aerobic exercise in order to receive fitness benefits.** This is similar to the myth that muscle weighs more than fat. While yes, it's true for most people who exercise that they typically burn more calories during aerobic exercise rather than anaerobic exercise, it's primarily due to the fact that they are spending more minutes performing aerobic than anaerobic exercise. In truth, we actually burn more calories per minute during high intensity anaerobic exercise, but because we cannot sustain it (the duration) when we add up the total calories burned during an hour or so of exercise the *total* is greater for the aerobic period because we performed more aerobic exercise than anaerobic exercise. That's why it's important to train and condition yourself to prolong your period of anaerobic-type exercises, resulting in more calories being burned per minute of exercise. Depending on the current level of fitness of an individual, one can derive both fitness and health benefits whether exercising for 5 minutes or 20 minutes. Let me show you how: Let's say you are 50 pounds overweight and completely unfit and decide to start walking to help you get exercising. Because you are not in the best of condition, you are only capable of walking for 10 minutes before you become totally exhausted and the distance you traveled is a little over a quarter of a mile. Every other day you walk, adding one to two minutes of duration each week, results in your walking longer and farther. Your eating habits remain exactly the same and at the end of one month, lo and behold, you weigh yourself and find you have lost a couple of pounds. In addition to having lost a few pounds, you now can walk for 15 minutes without needing to take a break and your speed has picked up to the point where you cover nearly a half a mile in that same 15 minutes, whereas just a mere month ago you could only cover half that distance in two-thirds the time (10 minutes). So, I ask you, did you derive fitness benefits from these jaunts even though you did not exercise or move for 20 minutes? Of course you did. We know this to be a fact and accurate because you were not able to walk 15 minutes when you first started out walking. In addition, you were not able to walk with the same intensity (speed) on day 1 as on day 30. What many people don't realize is that you need to start walking for 10 minutes in order to increase your time and lengthen your distance to 15 minutes and that half a mile. You could not have gone to 11, 12, 13, 14, and 15 minutes without going through the necessary steps of increasing your time.

One of the many wonderful and powerful things about exercise is that the benefits derived vary from person to person depending upon the current level of fitness and intensity at which the exercise is being performed. Now, a fit person who only walks for 10–15 minutes at the same speed or duration as the unfit individual would derive little or no fitness benefits and *would not* be able to lose weight unless taking in and consuming much fewer calories. This is a common behavior for millions of everyday exercisers and the main reason that they "plateau" or stop seeing or deriving benefits that are necessary in maintaining weight loss or improving their physique. Two and three years later, they're still walking at 3.5 miles per hour for 30 minutes. One of the positive things that comes with being overweight and unfit is that you can realize benefits from performing exercises with even low to moderate intensity. First of all, that's all your body and system is capable of. When you add up the calories being burned through exercise, depending on how often (frequency) you choose to walk that 10 minutes or more, 300 to 500 percent more calories are burned than when you used to exercise zero out of seven days!

Escape Route #27: We all want the Z in fitness and in life, but so few possess the patience and perseverance or see the logic to go A, B, C, D, E, and so on to that Z. That's why so many overweight and out-of-shape people don't even bother to begin to work out and exercise, because they think, *Why bother? I'm so out-of-shape that I can't do much, so why should I even start?*

Answer: **Myth.**

Fact or Myth #9: **Sit-ups are not an effective way of strengthening your abdominals and can actually hurt your back and do more harm than good.** You know, I can't for the life of me recall or remember the last time a boxing match, amateur or professional, was canceled because one of the boxers had developed back problems because of all the sit-ups he was doing in preparation for his fight, can you? I bet you also didn't know that bent-knee sit-ups are now a major component and rehabilitative exercise for recovering from back injuries and surgeries, did you? Not a crunch, a full bent-knee sit-up, my friend. They are not synonymous! Nine out of ten times when I ask a first-time client at Exude to do some sit-ups he/she immediately places his/her hands behind his/her neck, bringing his/her knees upward toward his/her chest, and proceeds to do a jerking limited-range-of-motion "crunch." "What the —— is that?" I ask. "That's not a sit-up, that's a crunch, and you're not even doing *that* correctly!" I exclaim. Then I demonstrate what I mean by a proper sit-up and ask him/her to do just one, and he/she can't even do *one* bent-knee sit-up. "That's pathetic," I say. "How many years have you been doing crunches and you cannot even do one simple sit-up?" And this is the typical response I get: "Everything I read says that sit-ups are bad for your back."

It's at this time that I need to explain myself again. Only this time I want to be miked up via satellite to the Times Square billboard and declare a state of emergency, so that I don't have to ever repeat myself another few thousand times and give the real lowdown concerning sit-ups. And this is what I would say: "When you lock your feet under a bed or bar and do sit-ups, then they are bad for your back because you are pulling and using more of your back than you are your abs. Here, let me show you." I then proceed to ask him/her to do a bent-knee sit-up again, only this time I am holding his/her feet down with my hands and poof like magic, he/she is able to do a few. See what I mean now? Sit-ups done properly can be a very effective exercise in strengthening your abs and back. "There are many muscle groups that a sit-up hits and works," I explain. "And there are different techniques and various degrees of intensity at which a bent-knee sit-up can be performed so as not to cause injury; you just haven't been taught them yet." If you are not capable of performing a bent-knee sit-up *without* straining your back and/or coming up and favoring one side of your body and I proceed to direct you to do a number of repetitions, then inevitably you'll hurt your back or some other region of your body. But was it the sit-up that was bad for you or was it more the case that the exercise I asked you to perform was too intense for your current level of fitness? Just as if I asked you to bench-press three hundred pounds and see if you could do one repetition and in doing so you arched your back and pulled it, was it the bench press exercise that injured you or the three hundred pounds being too much weight, thus too intense for your current level of fitness, that injured you? Suppose I asked you to bench-press one hundred pounds instead of three hundred pounds and you were able to perform fifteen repetitions? Do you get it now?"

Answer: **Myth**.

Fact or Myth #10: **If you genetically are preprogrammed to have large thighs or large arms, then there's not much you can do to alter it**. Yes, while it's true that you cannot do anything about your genetic makeup meaning that you have a propensity to hold extra fat or bulk up in certain regions of your body, it's not accurate that you can't do anything to alter it for the better. Your body type, current weight, and *type* of exercises you choose to do, coupled with the amount of weight/resistance, have far more of an impact than your genetics on streamlining your body. If you go to a gym or health club, the next time you go, take a look at the *size* of the butts and thighs of women coming out of a Spinning or step class. Did you notice that nine out of ten times, the instructor herself isn't exactly petite in these areas? Or how about the gals doing lunges holding dumbbells going around and in and out of the weight section of the gym with their trainer tailing behind pushing them to keep going? Yeah, keep going from a size 10 to a size 16, I say. It's all true. Remember. I am just the messenger, so don't shoot me.

The scary thing is when I ask these women (as I often do) when I visit a gym or health club what they think they're accomplishing while lunging, everyone responds by saying, "Firm and getting rid of my fat rear end."

"Oh, really"? I respond. "And how long have you been squatting and lunging?"

"Oh, not that long, about a year."

"I can tell it's really working," I say.

"What do you mean?" they shoot back (with a glance as well).

"What I mean is that you're wasting your time."

"How do you know?" they counter.

I then need to get very crafty and hit hard yet be sensitive, so I counterpunch with, "I'm not telling you that it isn't working; your body is telling you it isn't working. I'm just making you aware that it isn't working. Let me ask you something. If you had a skin rash and your doctor prescribed penicillin for you, two pills a day for thirty days, after which

> *Escape Route #28:* To avoid serious injury, it is far safer to do an exercise using less weight or resistance and performing multiple repetitions rather than perform the same exercise utilizing heavy weights or resistance and performing fewer repetitions. Once you get your muscles and joints stronger and you don't have to compromise form and alignment, then gradually increase the weight, and by doing so you will ensure safety and your body will be able to better absorb the benefits.

the skin rash did not get visibly better, would you ask for a refill, and keep taking it?"

"Of course not. I would get a second opinion and get a different prescription," they reply.

"Then why would you keep exercising the same and incorrect way *knowing* that your current fitness prescription is not helping you achieve your aesthetic goals?"

I have to say, though, that today either most of these women have become my clients or, the smart ones, have taken a step back and purchased one of my books and are now making positive steps in changing their body for the better. In life, and fitness is part of life, generally, people fear change.

I learned a long time ago, it's not enough to just say, "That's wrong," and end it there. You need to offer credible information and give examples in order to strike a chord and to drive home a point. Fitness is a very emotional topic with most people. That's why when our partner, parent, or sibling tells us to do something about our current state of fitness or that we have weight or eating issues, we tend to take it as a negative criticism rather than a genuine concern or caring.

Answer: **Myth.**

Fact or Myth #11: **The best time of the day to exercise is in the morning because it allows your body to burn calories throughout the day**. Actually, the best time of day to exercise is when your schedule allows you to be most consistent. Whether it's early A.M., midday, or early or late evening isn't as important as the actual act of working out. However, there are certain physiological and psychological advantages to exercising at different times of the day.

For instance, I have personally experienced that when I exercise early in the morning I am not as strong as when I work out in the late afternoon or early P.M. Also, when I perform a full-body routine in the early A.M. I'm tired throughout the entire day, yet when I only perform aerobic activity and abdominal exercises in the early A.M. I'm energized throughout the day. This fatigue is due to the fact that my heart has been at a resting pace for hours (six to eight) from sleeping the night before and when you do anaerobic exercise your heartbeat pounds harder and faster though your system has not totally woken up yet. I tend to exercise in the late afternoon or early evening because that's when my schedule allows me to be most consistent and I can still work afterward during the week. On weekends, I do work out in the morning but not very early (9:00 A.M.-ish), because if I don't get it done in the morning I will be too tired later from all my other activities: gardening, fishing, yard work, golfing, et cetera. On the other hand, my pal Neal prefers to work out in the very early morning (6:30 A.M.). And it doesn't get him tired like it does me. All of our bodies work on a clock that takes years to adjust or readjust to. The problem that some people may encounter is that their schedule dictates they exercise at one time of the day, yet their body clock where they are more alert does not match that particular time slot. This is not an impossible situation but takes much more motivation on your part to be consistent because your body is fighting against you and, let's face it, it could take some of the enjoyment out of it. If this is the case, don't despair, because with time your body clock will readjust itself; it's just going to take you a little more time for this amendment to become more and more comfortable. The most important thing is to pick the time slot when you are less apt to cancel, so you can establish consistency.

For those who need to exercise in the late P.M., that could keep you up past your normal bedtime and interrupt your sleep patterns, because it takes anywhere from four to six hours to allow your body to completely cool down to its normal core temperature, depending upon the intensity of your workout. So if you need to wake up and start your next day very early, try to exercise a bit earlier if this sleepiness is occurring. That's why I work out at about 5:00 to 7:00 P.M. during the week, so that my metabolism is revved up and I burn fat while I am sleeping. I typically start my downward spiral about 11:30, watching television, followed by reading, and falling asleep anywhere from 12:00 to 1:00 A.M., depending upon a number of factors, and wake up anywhere from 7:00 to 9:00 in the morning, depending on my commitments the next day. In the early morning is when I do my writing at home, because I am most alert mentally. By the time I get to the office and into the swing of things, I'm bombarded from all sides and can't focus on writing because my mind and body are in different modes.

There is no scientific evidence that exercising in the early A.M. or evening provides you with any advantage or disadvantage pertaining to weight loss and fitness.

I cannot tell you how often I observe people who "think" they're working out on their cell phones or chatting with their friends or partners or trainers. A major part and benefit of exercise extends far beyond just the physical gifts we receive. In fact, if you are exercising properly and focusing on only the task at hand your mind should be at complete rest, allowing you to relieve the stress in your life. You should not be "on" and should not be worrying about finances, family, love concerns, et cetera.

Escape Route #30: The best time to work out is when your schedule allows you to carve out three to five hours per week of pure uninterrupted time.

I always feel invigorated and energized yet calm after a good workout. My confidence is greater and I feel as if I can overcome any obstacle in life that is in my way. That's the goal and gift I want to give all of you reading this book, to experience *nirvana* each and every time you exercise!

Answer: **Myth.**

Fact or Myth #12: **Spas are an excellent way or means of helping you achieve and getting you on the right path for weight loss.** Do you know how many CEOs, businessmen and businesswomen, and others go away to these spas the same time each year to lose weight and "get back on track" with their weight-loss and eating habits? Well, obviously a lot, because spas are doing very well and I haven't read or heard of any of the major ones shutting down or going out of business despite our wonderful economy, have you? What's wrong with the following scenario? You're vastly overweight and enroll for a two-week stay at your favorite spa because in the past you have had success in losing 10 pounds and getting a jump start on losing weight and feeling better about yourself there. Well, the first thing that is blatantly wrong or "off" is that you are returning to the spa for the very same "fix" that didn't work the previous year or years. If it were so "great" or effective, you'd be writing and sending them a testimonial rather than forking over many thousands of dollars year after year, don't you think? It's as if a therapist gave you advice and you were sincere and honest with yourself and actually followed the advice and your problems remained unsolved or, in some cases, you took a step backward. Are you still going to keep your scheduled appointments and hand over that hundred dollars a session? Yet with weight loss and fitness you are blinded or maybe in denial that maybe, just perhaps, there might be a better way or more effective means to help you achieve your goals. In any event, you get my point. The main reason for your failure is because the environment and lifestyle you live in every day cannot and is not duplicated when you frequent the spa. Practically anyone can lose weight if he/she has a chef cooking healthy meals, has a structured exercise time with a trainer a few times a day, and gets out for walks or other activities at the spa; it's practically idiot-proof. What's not idiot-proof is when you come back home and you're commuting to and from work each day, shoving a bagel and coffee down your throat while driving or being driven to work, dealing with work stress, home life stress, and family issues, and have people clawing at you in every direction and you can hardly find the time and motivation necessary to eat correctly and exercise consistently and properly. Remember, weight loss is simple: calories in equal calories out. While at the spa, you are constantly moving, burning calories, eating sensibly, and exercising daily and the total number of calories you are burning up far exceeds your daily intake, thus you lose weight. But when you shift gears and come back to your everyday environment, your activity level drops, your food is not as carefully prepared, and before you know it the weight gain creeps up and you have gained all the weight you lost at the spa, plus more.

Answer: **Myth.**

Fact or Myth #13: **When your body hits a plateau, you need to constantly change and alter your fitness regimen in order to improve.** Based on this theory, ballet dancers and swimmers would not look as fit and trim as they do. They exercise practically the same way day after day. Are these ballet dancers and swimmers playing basketball and football or boxing a few days a week in combination with their daily fitness regimens? I don't think so. They do, however, cross-train and interval-train, which means incorporating different modes (types) of exercise combined with performing these exercises at different levels of intensity or speed for particular movements. The one and only downside about fitness is that as we become more fit, we *must* keep increasing the intensity at which we exercise in order to keep receiving the same health and fitness benefits as when we began our fitness regimen. The problem is that most people aren't educated in the proper techniques to keep increasing intensity within the same exact fitness routine and parameters in which they are currently exercising.

For instance, if you are 50 pounds overweight and walk a mile a day, after a month, as you have become more fit and lost, let's say, five to eight pounds, you are burning far fewer calories for that mile than when you first started walking, because the heavier we are, the more calories we burn no matter what we do, whether it is getting out of bed, bending over, walking a flight of steps, or walking to our car. Also, the energy expended in the beginning of your fitness walk is now far less after a month because your cardiovascular system and muscles are more fit than in the beginning. When you had first begun walking, it took you 30 minutes to walk that mile and your heart rate was 80 percent of your maximum heart rate (220 minus your age gives you your maximum heart rate; see chapter 4 for a complete description and heart rate chart). Now, one month later, your heart rate reaches and only requires you to use 60 percent of your maximum heart rate in order to walk that same mile. What this means numbers-wise is that you are working approximately 20 percent less than when you started, coupled with the fact that you are now lighter in weight so the amount of calories you are burning is considerably

> *Escape Route #32:* Before you start any weight-loss or fitness program, make sure it mimics your everyday environment and daily lifestyle—otherwise you will not be able to maintain consistency and thus will fail, time after time.

less than when you started out one month earlier. This is just one example of hundreds I could give you in regard to this topic, but it is perhaps the easiest to comprehend. You already know from reading this book that walking by itself is not fitness per se. I am just giving you a simple example that illustrates the fact that it is easy to see why one can plateau and it's not because you need to switch up your exercise routine in order to keep burning calories and to keep improving the way your body looks and performs. This plateau that most people refer to has more to do with current exercisers who perform the same exercise routine that they have been doing for some period of time but have not increased the intensity at which they are working.

Assuming that you are incorporating all five components within your daily fitness regimen, coupled with the fact that you are following the four phases of workout *and* exercising properly to reach your desired goals, there are a number of options and ways that you can prevent or alter this plateau. For instance, getting back to the 50-pound-overweight person who is now a month into his/her walking regimen, he/she can prevent pleateauing by increasing either the speed at which he/she walks or the duration (add 10 minutes, thus walking farther). Which is more effective? Actually, a combination of both is the most effective; however, the rule of thumb for first-time exercisers or out-of-shape individuals is to increase the duration rather than the speed, because then the risk of injury is far less. As you become more fit and your heart has been better conditioned, you are more apt to increase the speed but not the duration, because let's face it, are you going and do you have the time to walk for two hours a day? Highly doubtful! Everyday exercisers who are well conditioned can increase the speed, order of exercises, number of repetitions, and/or amount of weight or resistance used while exercising and take fewer breaks (active rests), or do interval training within the same exercise. For example, if you jog, crank up either the incline or speed for a short duration (two minutes or more), then bring it back down when you find you are starting to overtax your system, and then when you get your breath back crank it up again, and do a number of these intervals within your mode of exercise—hence the phrase *interval training*. Or you can cross-train, meaning add another mode (type) of exercise into your repertoire of exercises. If you normally just jog, walk, or run for your aerobic portion, try biking, jumping rope, or using an elliptical machine. Your heart and muscles are only used to performing and reacting to your current type of exercise and by adding a new exercise you will tax your system and hit other muscle groups that typically are not being worked during your normal exercise regimen. But the determining factor is the intensity at which you are working at, no matter which way you choose to exercise in order to prevent this plateau from occurring.

Answer: **Myth.**

Fact or Myth #14: **Only 25 percent of Americans exercise two to three times a week year-round.** Huh? Believe it or not, only 10 percent of the entire adult population (18 and older), exercise two to three times a week, year-round. And in my expert opinion, only 10 percent of that 10 percent are doing so in order to realize fitness, health, and aesthetic benefits. Scary, don't you think? It's no accident that over 60 percent of American children are obese or overweight, because that number mirrors the percentage of obese or overweight adults in this country. And it's not just an isolated problem here in America. Although we are a very overweight population, the people of many countries today are faced with the same and other health-related issues because of the lack of *proper* exercise that their population engages in daily. To further prove my point that only 10 percent of the existing 10 percent of current exercisers are receiving benefits: in the last 10 years, we have become 10 pounds heavier, yet health club and gym memberships have *doubled*. This can only mean either one of two things: either people are going to the health club or gym and not utilizing their time efficiently or they have signed up for memberships but are not going. It's really both, but more due to the fact that people are not going. And if they do get to the gym, they don't have a clue as to how to exercise in a fashion that gives them the results that they are searching for. Did you know that your heath club has 10 times the number of members that it could possibly service at any one time? Why is this so? It's for many reasons. But speaking frankly (as if I haven't been, right?), a typical large gym in any metropolis has a few thousand members. The most that the club can comfortably accommodate is about two hundred at any one time. That means that if only 20 percent of their 2000 members showed up at any one time (400 people), they would have to shut the doors after just a tenth of their members showed up to exercise on any given day. It's mind-boggling, isn't it? They are banking on the fact that you won't show up because if you do, they lose money. No rational person would join a gym or health club that had no room to comfortably accommodate him/her. Most people join health clubs and gyms for all the wrong reasons.

I suggest that if you are just starting out, don't like health clubs, have an incredibly hectic lifestyle, or simply don't feel comfortable in that type of setting, purchase a piece of aerobic equipment such as a bike or treadmill or elliptical, an exercise mat, and a weighted bar and jump rope and work out at home. Aside from the fact that you will have fewer

Escape Route #33: If you are highly motivated and have a clear understanding of how to exercise properly to meet your goals, then joining a health club or gym is the *right* move, if not, it's the *wrong* move.

distractions, you will be able to exercise whenever you want and your chances of maintaining consistency will be much better.

To make my point more convincing, when was the last time you joined a health club or gym and the salesperson sat you down and discussed a formidable game plan for you that took into consideration your lifestyle, medical and orthopedic limitations, current level of fitness, eating habits, current level of motivation, and all the other things that get in the way of you becoming consistent and thus successful in your quest for weight loss or to possess a fit body? Or does this sound more familiar: You got a tour of the club, were shown all the up-to-date fitness equipment, told of all the wonderful new and faddy classes now being offered, and offered the option to work with one of their trainers to go through an equipment orientation whose main objective was to get you to buy a package of generic-type exercise sessions?

Answer: **Myth.**

Fact or Myth #15: **If you have a bad back, or knees or suffer from diabetes and/or other ailments, you should limit the amount of exercise you are performing in order to avoid further complications.** These conditions are very common, especially among the older population. The fear of further injuring ourselves is greater than the motivation we possess, and I can certainly understand most people's apprehension. However, this is a clear case of naïveté. "Why should I even start to exercise when I don't even know what to do? What if I move too quickly or throw my back out again? I don't want to become bedridden again. It's too late anyway, I am sixty years old, vastly overweight, my life is practically over, so what's the use?"

Remember me telling you that there is a direct correlation between motivation and educating yourself about how to work out to reach your particular goals? Well, whether your goal is weight loss, toning, or gaining the knowledge of how to exercise despite a certain medical or orthopedic condition, it is no different. Read, ask questions of health professionals, go to clinics, and, basically, do whatever you need to do, including selling your soul, in order to create a clear path to making proper exercise a consistent part of your life. Otherwise, you will continue to live an unproductive life—mentally, physically, and spiritually! A common faux pas that many people make, especially after recovering from any type of surgery, is either go through rehab/physical therapy and then do nothing afterward or half-heartedly go through the motions of rehab/physical therapy and then do nothing.

You'd be surprised how many people suddenly stop doing anything

Escape Route #34: It's never too late to start exercising, because if you exercise properly for one year, the body reacts as if it has been exercising its entire life!

right after their rehab is finished. You need to stop feeling sorry for your-self, pick your butt up off the ground, and get moving! I don't need to tell you the advantages of proper exercise, especially if you suffer from diabetes, osteoporosis, or any other ailment. But I do need to tell you about the ramifications if you *don't* start exercising, especially if you are a diabetic. Basically, if you choose not to exercise and lose weight, you will be miserable, but it's your choice to be lazy. Obviously, it isn't a big enough priority for you to lose weight, strengthen your joints and mus-cles, and lower you medication; you'd rather be a walking time bomb, right?

Hey, I know it's not easy, especially if you are constantly in pain or un-comfortable. But Rome was not built in a day. Instead of thinking and fo-cusing on your pain and anguish, you need to channel your energy toward taking small, steady, and positive steps to get some weight off and strengthen your body. If I had to recommend *one* piece of equipment for those who suffer from most knee and back conditions or diabetes, it would be a *recumbent stationary bicycle*. It supports your back and it shouldn't bother your knees or back because of the angle at which your body is positioned. Start slowly with light resistance/tension for a few minutes and work up to 45 minutes. Once you have acclimated your body and system to biking then you can start to do other exercises and calisthenics. For combating osteoporosis, if you cannot walk or jog the recumbent bike is an excellent form of aerobic exercise combined with performing lower and upper body exercises with a 10-pound weighted bar. Whatever you choose to do, make sure that it falls within your fit-ness prescription from your attending physician or health care profes-sional in order to avoid any type of injury.

Answer: **Myth.**

Escape Route #35: The chief purpose of rehab and/or physical therapy is to get you mentally and physically prepared to start exercising in a safe and effective manner that will eventually get you to fully recover.

BEFORE YOU CAN FORM BET-

TER EATING AND EXERCISING

HABITS, YOU FIRST NEED TO

PROPERLY ORGANIZE

YOURSELF.

CHAPTER THREE

What You Need to Know and Do Before You Start Your Journey

Eating, Drinking, and Calories Consumed

So, you want to improve your eating habits and start to exercise properly and consistently, right? Your enthusiasm is there, you are committed and willing to take the necessary steps in order to do so, but before you launch into Mach 3 speed, there are a number of important factors to consider that are equally important in your quest for permanent weight loss. For instance, have you thought about and, more important, answered all of the following questions regarding your new and improved nutrition and exercise plan? Here are just a few things you need to figure out before you can become consistent and make smart decisions that will save you time and help avoid mistakes:

- Do you know how to lower your total caloric intake when you eat out so often?

- Do you know how to make healthy food choices for you and your family?

- When you're hungry between meals, are your snack choices smart ones?

- Before you start exercising have you figured out where you'll be working out: at home, the gym?

- What if you travel often? Will your fitness program travel well with you and will you have access to the same equipment while on the road?

So I've put together a check-off list to help you get organized on your road to everlasting weight loss.

First, though, I have restructured and renamed the Food Guide Pyramid as we know it today. Although most of the food groups to choose from are "healthy" choices, it would be nearly impossible to maintain eating that much food day in and day out. In addition, it is far too much food and calories to consume daily for 9 out of 10 people unless they are able to exercise two hours a day, seven days a week. Your new guide is called your **Food Index.** It's a much simpler version and will help guide you to choose and eat your meals based on the necessary groupings of food needed for proper nutrition. Remember to carefully monitor your portion size and the total amount of food you are consuming.

A major reason that people gain weight even though they are eating healthy is the total amount of food and beverages they consume. To help prevent this from occurring, you first have to have an idea of how much to eat, no matter what food group you select from. The total amount of calories you need to take in daily to maintain your current weight is a simple formula to remember: take your current weight and multiply it by 10–12, depending on how intense your activity/fitness habits are. Weight loss or weight gain is determined by two major factors: (1) calories in, calories out, and (2) your BMR, which dictates how much energy (calories) you expend during resting state. The more you exercise (properly and with the right intensity), the more efficient your BMR. So, a sedentary man who weighs 200 pounds should take in about two thousand calories to healthily maintain his current weight. If he exercises five times a week and expends 700 calories per exercise session, then he should on "paper" have a deficit of 3,500 calories for that week, which equals 1 pound of weight loss, provided that, of course, he did not increase his total weekly caloric intake of 14,000 calories (7×2000). Now let's take a different scenario for the 200-pound man. Instead of trying to lose weight by exercising, he decides to only "diet" to achieve a 1-pound weight loss for the week. That means he must take in a daily average of only 1,500 calories for that week ($3500 \div 7 = 500$), in order to lose that pound. But aside from the fact that it takes much more discipline to only consume 1,500 calories per day, that still doesn't guarantee that he will lose that pound, because as he chose to only "diet" his BMR may have slowed down enough so he will only lose one-half or three-quarters of a pound or no weight at all. This is why most people who try to lose weight only by cutting their food intake inevitably cannot keep it up and end up gaining the weight back plus more!

For example, if you are only allowed 1,500 calories a day and you happen to drink a soda or beer (approximately 150 calories) in addition to your calories allowed for that day, you now need to create a deficit of 150 calories the next day to just be back at your break-even level for the week. That means that you are now only allowed 1,350 calories for the next day, and that's if you only consume an extra 150 calories. Can you imagine if you ate a piece of cake or had some ice cream? You'd be allowed so few calories the next few days that you would be miserable, irritable, and depressed and possess little energy to function at your best at work, at home, and, yes, sexually. But if you get off course with your eating plan and you happen to be exercising, you can make up that 150 calories by performing an extra 10 minutes of exercise as well as improving your BMR all at once. Remember, losing weight is like balancing your checkbook: you can't (or shouldn't) write a check if you don't have enough funds to cover it. That's the power of exercise: it helps regulate your checkbook (your body), when you get off track. And let's face it: you *will* occasionally overeat or imbibe from time to time, but attempting to lose weight *strictly* by "dieting," with no exercise component, is clearly not the prudent choice.

A quick note here about my feelings about following *any* diet or eating plan that doesn't allow a certain food group or groups. The human body requires certain essential vitamins, minerals, and other vital nutrients for us to sustain a certain level of health and energy. Until the day comes when someone can medically or scientifically prove to me that our bodies don't require any of these essentials, then I cannot support any eating plan or diet that is too extreme. Besides, if we cannot overindulge in our favorite food or beverage every once in a while, what fun would life be anyway? That's why I have a hard time buying into a mostly high-protein/fat diet, a high-carbohydrate and low-fat diet, or any other severe combination ratio eating plans. Besides, I don't care how much willpower you think you may possess: if your body craves carbs, it will eventually need to be satisfied. And what's better, eating an occasional piece of bread and butter or small serving of ice cream or eating a whole loaf of bread and spread of butter or pigging out on a quart of ice cream? Based on this type of logic, then every single person who ever mixed proteins with starches and carbohydrates as a child growing up would have been overweight. It's funny, I grew up with a total of seven children sitting down to eat dinner each evening and I can't recall my mother announcing before dinner that because we were all gaining weight as a family there would be no more steak, potatoes, salad, and vegetables served together and there would no longer be pasta, meatballs, and bread and salad, either; from now on we could eat only the meatballs and salad— no pasta! How come no one out of the seven children had a weight problem as youths, despite these protein to carbohydrate combinations? I'll

Escape Route #36:
Weight loss is cumulative, it's not about eating or exercising well for a day here and a day there, just as weight gain is also cumulative; you don't *gain* weight with an occasional bad-eating day, if you can counter it with proper exercise.

tell you why: it's because of the portion size served to us combined with the fact that we were not allowed in the house either before or after dinner until we played outside for an hour or more, which ensured that we were burning enough calories consumed for that day!

Again, calories in equal calories out. These crazy diets and eating plans came about because in general most people don't have any self-control when it comes to eating and their idea of a portion is far larger than the recommended portion size. I hate to tell you, but whether you take in extra calories in the form of protein, carbs, fat, candy bars, carrots, or lettuce, you will still *gain* weight. The body doesn't discriminate between food groups. You may be healthier if you overeat with carrots rather than steak, but you will not be thinner, my friend. So, if you are currently following a specified eating plan or diet that is extreme in any way, pay attention to the total calories you are consuming; otherwise you could end up fatter when your goal is to become thinner!

That being said, here's the present Food Guide Pyramid, which you can compare to your new and easy-to-follow **Food Index** on the following pages.

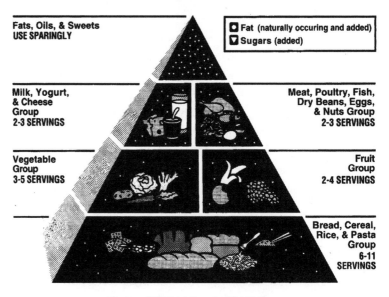

FOOD GUIDE PYRAMID
A GUIDE TO DAILY FOOD CHOICES

Fats, Oils, & Sweets
USE SPARINGLY

☐ Fat (naturally occuring and added)
☑ Sugars (added)

Milk, Yogurt,
& Cheese
Group
2-3 SERVINGS

Meat, Poultry, Fish,
Dry Beans, Eggs,
& Nuts Group
2-3 SERVINGS

Vegetable
Group
3-5 SERVINGS

Fruit
Group
2-4 SERVINGS

Bread, Cereal,
Rice, & Pasta
Group
6-11
SERVINGS

Source: U.S. Department of Agriculture

Your new Food Index for adults consists of the following groups, portion sizes, and servings:

GROUP I: BREAD, CEREAL, RICE AND PASTA GROUP *(3–5 Servings Daily)*	▪ 1 slice of bread or a small roll ▪ 1/2 cup cooked pasta, rice, or grain ▪ 1/2 cup starchy vegetables (corn, peas, or winter squash) ▪ 1 small potato or yam (1/2 cup mashed potato) ▪ 1/2 English muffin or a small bagel or hamburger/hot dog roll	▪ 3/4 cup unsweetened ready-to-eat cereal ▪ 1/2 cup bran cereal ▪ 1/4 cup Mueslix, low-fat granola, or Grape-Nuts cereal ▪ 1/2 cup cooked oatmeal ▪ 1/3 cup beans ▪ 3 cups popcorn
GROUP II: FRUIT GROUP *(4 Servings Daily)*	▪ 1 medium orange, apple, pear, plum, et cetera ▪ 1/2 medium banana ▪ 1 cup berries or melon	▪ 1/4 cup dried fruit ▪ 2 tablespoons raisins ▪ 1/2 cup fruit juice
GROUP III: VEGETABLE GROUP *(4 Servings Daily; salad doesn't count unless it is a salad with lettuce and other vegetables mixed in together)*	▪ 1/2 cup cut-up vegetables, raw or cooked ▪ 1 cup leafy green vegetables	▪ 1/2–3/4 cup vegetable juice with no sugar added
GROUP IV: MILK, YOGURT, AND CHEESE GROUP *(2–3 Servings Daily)*	▪ 1 cup milk, skim, low-fat, or whole ▪ 1 cup yogurt	▪ 1/2 cup cottage cheese ▪ 1/2 oz. cheese (choose low-fat varieties)

GROUP V: MEAT, POULTRY, FISH, DRY BEANS, AND EGGS GROUP (2–3 Servings Daily)	<ul><li>3 oz. cooked meat (3 ounces = size of a deck of cards)</li><li>1 egg</li></ul>	<ul><li>4–6 oz. fresh chicken, turkey, or fish</li></ul>
(For non-meat eaters the following foods are equivalent to 1 ounce of protein (7 grams of protein, 0-8 grams of fat):	<ul><li>1/4 cup cottage cheese</li><li>1 egg</li><li>1/2 cup beans</li></ul>	<ul><li>1/2 cup tofu</li><li>1 oz. cheese</li></ul>
GROUP VI: FATS AND OILS (2–3 Servings Daily)	<ul><li>1 teaspoon of oil, butter, or mayonnaise</li><li>1 tablespoon of reduced-fat butter or mayonnaise</li><li>1 tablespoon of cream cheese</li><li>1 tablespoon of vinaigrette salad dressing</li><li>2 teaspoons of peanut butter or any nut butter</li></ul>	<ul><li>6 cashews, almonds, or mixed nuts</li><li>4 pecans or walnuts</li><li>10 peanuts</li><li>1/8 medium avocado</li><li>8 medium olives</li></ul>
GROUP VII: DESSERTS (No more than 2 Servings per Week)	<ul><li>1/2 cup ice cream</li><li>1 small ice-cream sandwich</li><li>1 small piece of cake (3 x 3 inches)</li></ul>	<ul><li>1 cup fresh strawberries</li></ul>

**Please Note: Avoid saturated fats whenever possible and remember, *all* fats contain more calories than proteins or carbohydrates, so careful monitoring of the amount of fats you consume will help you lose weight and/or maintain your current weight. Also, try to avoid food with high sugar content. Aside from being unhealthy, a diet high in sugar has loads of calories but contains few nutrients.

You'll notice I separated out the fat, oils, and sweets from one another. The present Food Guide Pyramid says to use these sparingly. What does that mean? Based on that phrasing, one could eat a little dessert seven days a week and, in your mind, be eating dessert sparingly. It's important to note here that when eating daily one must keep a log either by memory or writing down certain foods and the quantity consumed in order to properly manage caloric intake. For example, if you ate a large Danish and coffee for breakfast one morning, you probably consumed a minimum of 750 calories. If you weigh 150 pounds, then you only can consume approximately 1,500 calories for the entire day *without* gaining weight for that particular day. Now you must be very careful and choose the remaining 750 calories or so from all the other food groups *without* exceeding 1,500 calories. Aside from the fact that you chose to eat a dessert as a meal, try to remember what my mother always said to us while growing up: "Dessert is a *treat,* not a treatment!" Unfortunately, when the average person eats this way, he/she isn't fine-tuned enough or disciplined and knowledgeable enough to eat properly for the remainder of that day so you will likely gain weight for that particular Danish-eating day. This is a good example of how you need to pick and choose your calories wisely. This also takes many months and sometimes years to master. Too often, people don't realize how much food and the quality of foods they select are doing more harm than good, so be aware of *everything* you take in when trying to lose or maintain your current weight.

The upside to all of this of course is you always have your fitness regimen in your back pocket, sort of your trump card to counter your poor-eating days, which will allow you to at least not gain weight if you exercise intensely and often enough. But don't abuse this privilege, because it is only an insurance policy against gaining weight, not a sensible approach, and virtually impossible for long-term weight loss, which, don't forget, is your ultimate goal.

Now that you have a better idea as to how much food and which food groups to make smarter choices with, you can start to organize yourself and prepare ahead of time, which will ensure permanent weight loss. Here are some things for you to consider.

Your Waistline Check-Off List

Are you single, married, living with someone, or do you have children? Your current environment *dictates* your eating lifestyle and eating habits that you will need to adjust to as you start cutting calories. When and where do you do most of your eating? Are you prepared and capable of eating properly despite the fact that you may:

- **DINE OUT OFTEN?** There are a lot of hidden calories you need to be aware of when eating out: sauces, dressings, oils that your food are cooked in, and portion size. When ordering, ask for all of your food to be grilled and not fried, all sauces and dressings on the side. Share a full meal or, if dining alone, ask for a half-portion. Have seafood or salad as your appetizer, and avoid heavy broths and cream-type soups, which contain tons of calories. If you must, share dessert or order some low-calorie fruit such as strawberries without whipped cream!

- **TRAVEL?** Even if you travel first-class, whether it be via train, bus, or plane, most of the food served is highly processed and full of hidden sugars and saturated/hydrogenated fats. And don't wait till you get to the train or bus station or airport to buy from the fast-food selections; those are just as bad for you. Before you travel, either food shop ahead of time and prepare the number of meals you'll need for the trip or go to a health-food restaurant or deli that makes fresh already-prepared food for you to select from. Also, take plenty of fruit; it is a great filler food between meals that is typically lower in calories, with only trace amounts of fat. Avoid diet-type beverages, as they will dehydrate you if they contain caffeine as well as bloat you and contain virtually no nutritional value. And don't forget to drink plenty of water.

- **DO THE FOOD SHOPPING FOR A NOT ALWAYS NUTRITION-MINDED FAMILY?** Make a list *before* you go to the market. Statistics prove that when you have an itemized list, not only will you make smarter food choices but you will buy less food as well, which will save you money. Do not allow your children to grab their favorite sweets and sugar-coated cereals and place them in the shopping cart when your back is turned. Allow some leeway, but be firm—*no* means no—and explain to them why your choice is better in the long run for them than their selection of empty calories. Limit the amount of soda you buy and purchase desserts such as small ice-cream sandwiches rather than ice cream in tubs. Make sure you have a salad and three vegetables plus your selection of meat, fish, or poultry with each dinner. Also, remember to drink 32–64 ounces of water every day. Drinking water helps keep you full and cuts down on overeating. Have plenty of low-calorie and low-fat snacks handy for your children. And yes, drink milk unless, of course, you're allergic; it's good for you and your children. If your child's menu for lunch is inadequate from a nutritional point of view, make lunch for them to take to school and give them money to buy milk or a natural fruit juice.

- **HAVE SPECIAL DIETARY NEEDS?** Whether you are a vegetarian, allergic to certain foods, or simply a finicky or picky eater, it's especially important for you to do your research to secure places where you can have easy access to your food choices. And for those of you with any kind of special dietary needs so that your daily food intake is essential to your well-being, such as diabetics, you really need to prepare ahead and assume that virtually no food establishment will be able to satisfy your dietary needs, so please keep this in mind, especially when traveling.

THE USE OF VITAMIN SUPPLEMENTS

Since we can't all eat perfectly day in and day out, I am a big proponent of vitamins. To help ensure that we consume adequate amounts of all the essential nutrients, a government-sponsored organization called the Food and Nutrition Board of the National Research Council periodically establishes *Recommended Dietary Allowances,* or RDAs, of certain nutrients to be used as "standards to serve as a goal for good nutrition." (See page 46.) These numbers are only estimates of the body's need for a particular nutrient plus an extra safety margin meant to account for variability between individuals. Some experts believe that these RDAs are inadequate because they only refer to healthy individuals and do not address the special nutritional needs of the ill, as certain sicknesses and numerous medications greatly affect the way our bodies absorb and utilize nutrients, which can often *increase* our body's nutritional requirements. In addition, the RDAs do not take into affect lifestyle factors such as smoking, drinking, stress, exercise, et cetera.

In theory, if we eat properly we can ingest most or all of the nutrients needed to meet the RDA requirements. But in reality, today's highly processed foods and our stressed and rushed environment leave few of us time to consume the foods we should. The role of vitamins and supplements is not to be substituted for good nutrition *but* to bolster weak areas of a fairly adequate eating regimen. The combination of taking certain vitamins and supplements and eating well will ensure that you're getting the essential vitamins and minerals for optimum health.

But before you ingest any vitamins or supplements, I highly recommend checking with your doctor and asking him/her whether to take a daily multivitamin and mineral, vitamin B complex, vitamin C complex, antioxidant, or any other vitamin or supplement. And here's another tip you can do to ensure eating better for five months or more a year, depending where you live and its climate; start an organic vegetable garden. It will save you money on fresh produce and provide a great activity and gardening is something the whole family can enjoy doing together. In addition, your produce will be far more beneficial to you in terms of the vitamins ingested than store-bought produce.

Factors That Affect Weight Gain

Another reason that many people gain weight who live in areas where there are changes in seasons and truly cold winter months, is because activity level drops considerably during these three to four months. This is one of the most common reasons that people gain weight during the winter months, because even if they don't *increase* their caloric intake,

Recommended Dietary Allowances

Nutrient Fat-soluble Vitamins	Men RDA	Women RDA
Vitamin A (RE, I RE = I micro gm = 3.33 IU)	1,000	800
Beta-carotene (mg)	N/A	N/A
Vitamin D (micro gm, 1 microgram = 40 IU)	5	5
Vitamin E (IU, 1 IU alpha tocopherol equivalent to 1 mg alpha tocopherol)	10	8
Vitamin K (mg)	80	65
Water-soluble Vitamins		
Vitamin C (mg)	60	60
Vitamin B12 (mg)	2	2
Folic acid (micro gm)	200	180
Niacin (mg)	15	15
Pyridoxine (B6) (mg)	2	1.6
Riboflavin (B2) (mg)	1.4	1.2
Thiamin (B1) (mg)	1.2	1
Minerals		
Boron (mg)	N/A	N/A
Calcium (mg)	800	800
Chromium (micro gm)	50–200	50–200
Copper (mg)	1.5–3	1.5–3
Iodine (micro gm)	150	150
Iron (mg)	10	15
Magnesium (mg)	350	280
Manganese (mg)	2–5	2–5
Phosphorous (mg)	800	800
Potassium (mg)	99	99
Selenium (micro gm)	70	55
Sodium (mg)	500	500
Zinc (mg)	15	12

they burn up fewer calories during the cold months than the warmer months when during the week and weekends they enjoy their favorite sport or leisure activity. For instance, let's say you garden or walk the golf course for two hours twice a week. The average 150-pound person will burn approximately 320–360 calories per hour during these activities, representing a total caloric expenditure of 320×2 (hours) $\times 2$(days) = 1280–1440 calories each week. So if you are inactive for four months (about eighteen weeks) and you don't change your caloric intake at all, you consume an extra 18×1280–1440 = 23,040–25,920 calories, divided by 3,500 calories, which represent 1 pound, meaning that during those four months of hibernating you will gain 6.6–7.4 pounds! In order to avoid weight gain during these four months, you need to either (1) exercise more often, (2) cut your normal daily intake of calories, or (3) choose an activity that burns the same amount of calories during these four months as during the warmer months. Most people don't even realize why they gain weight during the winter, but now you have a very clear picture as to why so that you can make adjustments during this time frame; be conscious of and avoid the traps and pitfalls and prepare ahead during these more inactive cold winter months.

BMR

Throughout this book and elsewhere, the term *Basal Metabolic Rate (BMR)* is frequently used. We quite often read and hear how it's important to raise or increase your BMR and, by doing so, increase the amount of calories that you can burn throughout the day. Here I've put together in layman's terms what exactly BMR is and how it affects the number of calories that we burn during a typical day.

Your BMR is the number of calories you will burn in a 24-hour period in a basal (or lying) position but not sleeping. It accounts for 50 to 75 percent of your daily caloric expenditure. *Metabolism* is the body's process of converting food into energy to keep the body running and fuel daily activities. Your resting metabolic rate represents the number of calories your body burns to maintain vital body functions (heart rate, brain function, breathing). Most people understand metabolism as how slowly or quickly their bodies burn calories. Unfortunately, they don't understand how important it is for successful weight management. Weight management is a matter of simple arithmetic—balancing the number of calories in against the number of calories out. If you know how many calories you're burning (you caloric budget), you know how many calories you can eat to meet your weight management goals.

Muscle Consumes Calories

Because muscle burns calories, and body fat very few, the more lean muscle mass in your body and the lower the percentage of fat the more calories you will burn during physical activity. This also means you will burn more calories when you are sitting in a chair, reading a book, or even sleeping! When people diet, especially when they are not also exercising, they lose weight but often sacrifice muscle mass. This is because most diets provide too few calories. Calorie restriction can lead to muscle wasting, which leads to decreased metabolism. Severely restrictive diets can reduce your metabolic rate by up to 50 percent. This is, in part, why exercise is necessary, and not just any exercise, but a full-body fitness routine that includes aerobic and strengthening exercises, for losing and maintaining weight. We must exercise in this manner with the proper intensity in order to maintain muscle and bone density, thus boosting our metabolism.

HOW TO BURN MORE CALORIES

Eating: Digestion accounts for approximately 10 percent of the calories you use to process the food you consume. Each time you eat, your body uses energy to break down the food. When you eat small meals throughout the day, your body burns more calories than when you eat one big meal. Think of your metabolism as a fire. If you throw small meals (kindling) in every few hours your fire will burn better than if you throw one big meal (one big log) in once a day. In effect, eating on a regular basis helps you burn calories, provided that you don't overeat.

Physical Activity: When many people think of burning calories, they think only of vigorous exercise, such as running or taking a Spin class. However it is important to realize that all physical activity burns calories. Physical activity is the most important component of caloric expenditure that you have full control of. Anywhere from 15 to 40 percent of the calories you burn come from all of the various activities you perform throughout the day.

HOW TO DETERMINE YOUR BMR

The following formulas will help you calculate your approximate BMR. There are different formulas for men and women because men, as a fact of life, start out with more muscle mass than women and therefore burn more calories through their basal metabolism.

MEN: $66 + (13.7 \times W) + (5 \times H) - (6.8 \times A) = BMR$
WOMEN: $655 + (9.6 \times W) + (1.7 \times H) - (4.7 \times A) = BMR$

(W = Weight in kg. H = Height in cm. A = Age in years.)
To convert pounds to kg.: weight in lbs. divided by 2.2.
To convert inches to centimeters: height in inches times 2.54.

PLEASE NOTE: For your individualized eating plans and fitness regimens for weight loss, please turn to the chapter that applies to your weight reduction goals. (Chapters 5–8).

Fitness and Exercise

When I use the words *proper exercise,* as I do throughout this book, what goes through your mind? Do you have any idea what I mean? Well, I can tell you that it's not about going out for a leisurely stroll or walk. Nor is it about just taking a yoga class. Not that walking or yoga can't be *part* of your exercise regimen, but by itself such an activity will not help you in your quest for weight loss. Keep in mind I am only interested in the exercises that are the most effective in helping you lose weight, not those that merely make you "feel better." The reality of the situation is that you can't feel better unless you start losing weight. We only have a limited time each week to devote to our fitness program, and too often many people don't prioritize their exercise time effectively. The average person has about an hour a day five days a week that he/she can realistically devote to exercising. In that hour, you need to warm up, stretch, work out vigorously, and finally cool down. You also need to hit all five components during that hour: cardiovascular conditioning, muscle endurance, muscle strength, flexibility, and body ratio. You also need to exercise with the right intensity based on your current level of exercise coupled with the right type of exercises to achieve weight loss, meaning you need the correct percentage of aerobic and anaerobic exercise in order for that weight loss to occur. And you think you have time to fool around and take a leisurely walk and receive credit for exercising properly?

As I have said in *all* of my previous books and columns, which has since been medically substantiated, there are virtually very few health and minimal fitness benefits to most passive activities/exercises. The true reason is because when the average person performs any of these leisure activities, the intensity is not enough or sustained long enough for his/her body and system to benefit from it. That's why they're called *leisure* activities. And there is nothing wrong with engaging in and enjoying these activities or sports. The problem is, we are *substituting* them for proper fitness and they are not synonymous. It's not your fault, though. For many years the surgeon general and other medical-associated watchdogs have been telling us inaccurate facts, such as washing your car for 45 minutes or doing housework for 30 minutes or cutting your lawn for 30 minutes or so will adequately benefit you. Today, after years of study, literally thousands of people who did these or other related activities have been found to be just as fat or unfit as their contemporaries who did little or no such activity.

Escape Route #37: Walk for fun, not for fitness.

Your Fitness Check-Off List

GET A PHYSICAL

Whether you are 18, 30, 60, or older, get a full physical and stress test! You want to make sure that all cylinders are running properly *before* you start working out. In addition, if you are on any medication, especially any beta-blockers, you want to ask your doctor or health professional about your maximum heart rate and ask him/her for parameters concerning your intensity, et cetera. Also, for those who are suffering from any kind of orthopedic condition such as bad knees or bad back, ask your specialist if walking or biking is OK with your current condition. You don't want to go out and buy a treadmill, for instance, if you cannot walk or slow jog *without* putting undue stress on your joints.

WHAT YOU'LL NEED

One of the most important factors in becoming fit, staying fit, and maintaining consistent weight loss is where you'll be exercising and working out. For the purposes of this program you will need access to only a few pieces of fitness equipment. Specifically, you will be using: (1) a recumbent stationary bike, rebounder, treadmill, or you will be walking outside for your warming up, cooling down, and aerobic component of your workouts, (2) a firm exercise mat to do your calisthenics, (3) a lightweight two- or four-pound Collapsible Aerobic Toning Bar, and (4) a speed jump rope for those who are medically and orthopedically sound to do so. If you are a member of a gym or health club, they typically will have everything listed here except for the aerobic toning bar and/or a speed jump rope. If this is the case, you can log onto www.exude.com to purchase any piece of fitness equipment that you will need. The total square feet and exercise space required for all of your workouts is very small, about six feet by six feet. If you don't currently belong to a gym or club, I would seriously consider investing in this equipment for home use, because then you will have access twenty-four/seven, and without the hassle of waiting to use a bike or treadmill or feeling uncomfortable or self-conscious exercising in front of others. When purchasing a recumbent bike, look for a manual rather than electronic version, because there are two main advantages to manual bikes: (1) cost, as manual bikes are far less expensive, and (2) flexibility, as most electronic bikes are preset to resistance/tension levels that cannot be adjusted any lower and the setting is too high for most people starting out, which may hurt your knees and/or bulk you up instead of trimming you down, which of course is your goal.

BLOCKING OUT TIME

Get a weekly planner and each Friday jot down and schedule the days for the following Monday–Sunday that you can block out one hour toward your fitness and weight-loss regimen. The reason that you want to do this is because if you cannot work out on any particular day you can easily adjust and, wherever possible, change your days/times because you have your entire weekly schedule right in front of you. *Don't* wait for the week that you are currently in to pick and choose when you'll be exercising; it's too late and too many other constraints will prevent you from working out. And please don't tell me or, more important, yourself that you don't have enough time. (1) You control your own life and scheduling, and (2) make your exercise appointment a priority and treat it as if it were the biggest business appointment in your life!

The Four Essential Phases of Every Workout

Each and every time you exercise you need to follow a certain protocol that ensures you'll receive *all* the benefits of fitness as well as improving your health, increasing your fitness level, and help you lose weight. In addition, by following the four phases will lower your risk of muscle soreness and/or injury and will allow your body and system to absorb the stress and shock so that physiologically and psychologically you're not over-taxed. I call the four phases of a workout the Bible of fitness, because there are no deviations allowed and all four phases have been proven medically and scientifically to allow our bodies to change for the better faster than if we ignore one or more phases. To further motivate you to pay attention to and actually complete the four phases, think of this: tests show that if two people exercise the same way, the individual who follows the four phases not only looks better aesthetically but also has fewer injuries and is more fit than the individual who chooses to ignore performing the four phases during each and every workout. That being said, here are the four phases in the exact order for you to follow when you begin exercising.

Escape Route #38: A manual recumbent bike is the best piece of aerobic fitness equipment you can utilize for weight loss! Aside from the fact that it supports your back and knees, the speed at which you can pedal (RPMs) is so much faster than the speed you can walk *without* causing discomfort to your knees and/or back—which results in burning more calories, of course.

Escape Route #39: If you don't find time for exercise, sooner or later you will have to find time for sickness.

PHASE I: THE WARM-UP

Warming up has many purposes: it provides your entire body a smooth transition from the resting state to the higher level of energy expenditure and effort you experience in the main part of your workout; it raises your heart rate from its resting state gradually and safely in order to prepare your heart for more demanding activity; and it prepares your body physiologically and your state of mind psychologically for physical performance, not only to improve performance but also to lessen the possibility of injury. Warming up raises both the general body and the deep muscle temperatures and stretches collagenous tissues, which permits greater flexibility. It also increases your physical working capacity during your workout.

Put another way, think of starting a car that needs to be warmed up early in the morning when it's freezing outside and trying to pull away from the curb as soon as you start your engine. What happens? The car may start choking and misfiring and eventually stall out. Well, the same thing happens to your body when you don't warm it up before you start exercising. Men are guiltier than women of not warming up and stretching before they begin their workouts. When I travel and visit gyms, I cringe when I am sitting on my stationary bike warming up and almost every single guy who walks into the gym goes immediately to the weights and starts pumping away *without* any warm-up or stretching. If they only knew what harm they were doing to their bodies, perhaps they would take stock and change their bad habits. And these are the same guys who slam the weights, grunt and growl, and are more interested in looking at themselves in the mirror than performing the exercise with proper form, utilizing the mirror as their coach rather than for their ego. You know the type—they have peglike legs and a big upper body and typically have a gut. Trust me, buddy, the ladies are not looking at your biceps; they are laughing at how ridiculous and uneven your body looks.

A proper warm-up takes anywhere from 5 to 15 minutes, depending on how fast your body takes to feel loose and start to break a steady sweat. Aerobic exercise such as walking, slow jogging, stationary biking, walking in place, using an elliptical machine or cross trainer, and rowing are all good examples. The colder the weather, the longer your warm-up should be. The intensity (how hard you are working) should be of sufficient duration and intensity without developing marked fatigue. If you are just starting out, a stationary bike is best for warming up, riding it with minimal resistance. This raises your heart rate more safely than treadmilling, because you are only using about 50 percent of your body weight, unlike on a treadmill, where you are using your entire body weight.

For those who are looking to lose weight and mass, your warm-up will be considerably longer in duration (time). You also will be burning lots of calories during this warm-up phase, as you'll be doing a combination warm-up/aerobic portion all in one. As you turn to the chapter based on your weight-loss goals, you will find that your warm-up phase will be 20–30 minutes in length because of the fact that you need that extra time of performing aerobic exercise to aid you in shedding those extra pounds.

After you have completed your warm-up, you can now stretch, but don't allow more than 5–10 minutes to elapse between the end of your warm-up and performing your exercises, known as your *workload* phase.

PHASE II: STRETCHING

Most people, especially men, do not possess great flexibility. And even though genetics do play a role in flexibility, *everyone* can increase their flexibility if they learn the correct techniques and stretch for a few minutes each and every time *before* they begin exercising. The main reason for lack of flexibility is the fact that for many years of either being sedentary or while exercising a person never took the time to stretch because of either lack of knowledge or not realizing the importance of possessing good flexibility. In addition, by not stretching you will injure yourself more often, will not burn as many calories during your workouts as those who possess good flexibility, will put undue stress on your joints and always be sore, especially in your back region, and will not be able to increase your range of motion with any exercise you perform. Of all the major muscles to focus on and improve flexibility in, your *hamstrings,* which are located behind your legs, are the most important. In short, having good hamstring flexibility is your insurance policy for possessing and maintaining a healthy back for the rest of your life. I am always amazed by the number of clients who come to us for fitness advice and have never stretched before exercising, and the sad part is that most of these people have actually worked with personal trainers in the past!

The other main reason that people don't stretch, besides the fact that they loathe it, is because they have never been exposed or taught to do a simple three-to-four-minute full-body stretch routine that can be performed without assistance from another. Remember, there is a direct correlation between motivation and knowing what to do, and that applies to stretching as well. At the beginning of each exercise program based on your weight-loss goals, there is an easy-to-follow stretch routine for you to follow. No matter how uncomfortable or how much you hate it, do it anyway! One important tip to remember while stretching is to *never* bounce while stretching. Always hold the stretch and breath nor-

> *Escape Route #40:* Nine out of ten people who possess poor hamstring flexibility have either low-back pain or weak lower abdominal muscles.

mally and don't hold your breath or frown. Be relaxed, and with time you will increase flexibility throughout your entire body in 30 days or less.

PHASE III: THE WORKLOAD

Now that you've properly warmed up and stretched, you can start the workload phase of your workout. This is where synergy comes in—the parts together are far more powerful than the individual parts by themselves. When your body is properly prepared by having been lubricated, you can exercise with the proper intensity so that you are burning the most amount of calories possible during this, your workload phase. It is here that you rev up your speed, increase your number of repetitions, and perform exercises for your upper body, midsection, and lower body. Your workload is a menu of exercises that comprise your actual "workout" and is determined by: (1) your medical and orthopedic constraints (if any), (2) your goals: losing weight versus toning, and (3) your current level of fitness. Each exercise program I've designed for all the weight-loss categories is from 40 to 60 minutes in length, depending upon your current level of fitness. One of the biggest mistakes people make when starting out an exercise program is not taking into consideration their lifestyle and time constraints *before* they begin to work out.

Exercising an hour each time, five days a week, 48/52 weeks is more effective than two hours one or two days per week for that same year. In other words, frequency is your main objective when trying to lose weight and mass.

Since your *primary* goal is to lose weight and mass, your workload will primarily be *aerobic-type* exercises performed with low to moderate resistance/tension and at a high speed (RPMs). As you know by now after reading chapter 2, the heavier you are, the lighter the resistance/tension or weight to use will help trim you down. In case you ever forget or are resistant to believing me, all you need to do is think about the examples I've given you, specifically the bodies of marathon runners, triathletes, cross-country skiers, and swimmers. They are lean and more streamlined than their counterparts because of the fact that they perform more *aerobic-type* exercise and their training regimen is such for that to occur.

As you lose more weight, you can gradually add more tension/resistance and weight to all of your exercises, but not until you are happy with the *size and weight* of your body. This is very critical for your success, so please listen and follow your fitness prescription exactly as outlined, with no deviations.

Aerobic is defined as sustained, rhythmic large-muscle activity that does not require more than a low or moderate intensity (energy) level and can be performed continuously (without a break) without undue respiratory discomfort. For the purpose of weight loss, aerobic exercise is primarily used for improving your cardiovascular system *and* to take off weight and mass. Based on your current level of fitness, you may be able to sustain that activity for 2, 5, 10, 20, or 30 minutes or more. For those of you who are vastly overweight and/or out-of-shape, don't despair if you can initially only do a few minutes of aerobic exercise before you become fatigued, because the beautiful thing about exercise is that it is all relevant to the current condition of the subject. To be exact, if you are an unconditioned individual and all you can do is 5 minutes of stationary biking before you need to *physically* stop, as long as you taxed your cardiovascular system you have received the same fitness and health benefits as perhaps I receive by performing that same *exact* exercise for 20 minutes or more. This is important for you to realize, especially if you wonder why you should even bother to start exercising if you can do only a few minutes. This principle applies to *all* types of exercises; it is not just limited to aerobic exercise. For instance, if you can only do 1–3 modified push-ups (on your knees rather than your toes), you taxed your system just as much as I taxed mine if I performed 25 push-ups. The difference is I burned more calories because of the amount of time and number of repetitions I performed were greater, but you will still have benefited.

The key to building up muscle endurance, strength, and a more efficient cardiovascular system is frequency (how many times you perform your exercises per week) and slowly adding either duration (time) and/or repetitions.

For weight loss, adding resistance is not advisable for a few reasons: (1) the more resistance, the higher your heart rate goes, (2) the more resistance, the faster your muscles fatigue, and (3) the more resistance, the bulkier you will get. Remember, you cannot convert fat to muscle (review chapter 2). If you slowly add time (duration), let's say a minute or two each week to your aerobic exercise, and add one or two repetitions each two weeks to your push-ups, soon you will be on your way to reaching higher numbers, because you are more fit and as a result will burn more calories as well as raise your BMR.

One last thought about *aerobic* exercise: Because you are overweight, it is critical that the type of aerobic exercise you choose does not bulk up your legs, hips, or buttocks. When you have extra fat in any region of your body and you apply moderate to high tension/resistance to that area, you will add size rather than lose mass. Aerobic exercises such as Spinning, step classes, stair climbing, walking, and jogging on an incline, and using ellipticals with high resistance for both upper and lower body are no-nos for losing mass! Although you will burn calories performing these types of exercises, the rate at which you will build muscle can be greater than the rate at which you are burning calories.

Conversely, *anaerobic* exercise is defined as exercising "without the presence of oxygen." The term *without oxygen* refers to your body's inability to take in as much oxygen as it needs during anaerobic exercise. This is because during anaerobic exercise your heart rate zooms upward, preventing your body from taking in oxygen as readily. Examples of anaerobic exercise include weight lifting, sit-ups, pull- and chin-ups, push-ups, squats, lunges, running up a flight of stairs, running a 100-yard dash, shoveling snow, and downhill skiing. In short, any stop-and-go activity that requires short bursts of energy to perform. "Any form of exercise that requires a break" is a good way to define and understand anaerobic exercise. Your body requires a break because your heart rate is closer to maximum than during aerobic exercise, when it beats at a lower rate and does not require you to stop to get your breath. Some exercises and sports are a combination of both aerobic and anaerobic exercise, such as full-court basketball, hockey, and a long singles tennis match.

Anaerobic exercise is primarily used for *toning* and building muscle. Although it is important when trying to lose weight to do a combination of aerobic and anaerobic exercise, aerobic exercise takes precedence over anaerobic exercise because you cannot firm fat and you don't want to build muscle under the fat, which will *increase the size* of the region of the body being worked. As you lose more weight, you can *slowly* increase the amount of anaerobic exercise into your workload portion of your exercise routine. But it's important to note that to keep that weight off that you've lost and to maintain your current weight or lose even more, the percentage of *anaerobic* exercise will *never* exceed the amount of aerobic exercise you'll be performing during workouts for the rest of your life. So, the rule of thumb is simple: the heavier you are, the more aerobic exercise you need, and the thinner you are, the more anaerobic exercise you need in order to possess a balanced and symmetrical body.

When just starting out or if you are out-of-shape, some aerobic exercises "act" *anaerobically.* For instance, although jogging is considered aerobic exercise, if you jog at six miles per hour and your cardiovascular system is not conditioned enough to take that intensity, your heart rate will zoom to a point in a minute or so when you will have to either stop or slow down in order to take in oxygen so that you can continue jogging. That's why it's important to warm up and stretch *before* you start exercising intensely, because your chances of a heart attack or injury are lessened. If you do not warm up, your heart rate will go from, let's say,

Escape Route #42:
When performing aerobic exercise, of the two, in order to reduce size, speed (RPMs) is your friend and resistance/tension is your enemy.

a resting heart rate of 80 Beats Per Minute (BPM) to 150 BPM in a matter of one minute, rather than allowing your heart to make small, gradual jumps of 80–90–100–120–130–150, and so forth. The shock to your system is far less because you have properly warmed up and stretched.

The type of training you choose, *endurance* versus *strength,* is the major factor that allows you to shed weight or gain unwanted size. Endurance-type exercises add more to your cardiorespiratory reserves. Conversely, strength-type exercises are not as effective for adding to your long-term aerobic capacity. Both types are forms of **anaerobic** exercise. An example of endurance-type exercise is lifting or moving a light-to-moderate-weight object many times (repetitions) *without* having to rest or stop. Some examples of endurance-type exercises are calisthenics, such as sit-ups, leg lifts, jumping jacks, squat thrusts, and lifting a light weight five pounds for 50–100 repetitions without resting.

Strength training requires moving a heavy weight/object only a few times (repetitions). Examples of strength training include bench presses, squats, leg presses, and shoulder presses with heavy weights, with no more than 8–12 repetitions. One great benefit of endurance-type exercises is that they protect your body from injury. The more fatigued you are, the more susceptible you are to injury. When you put physical demands on your body that it cannot sustain, something has to give. Visually, think of a ballet dancer or swimmer's body (endurance-type exercisers), versus a weight lifter, speed skater, sprinter, or typical football player's body (strength-type exercisers).

As I've mentioned earlier, we actually burn *more* calories during anaerobic exercise than we do while performing aerobic exercise per second of time, but most exercisers cannot sustain their anaerobic movements long enough to burn as many total calories as they do while exercising aerobically. And it's the total amount of calories used during your exercise regimen that is the most important factor in creating a deficit of calories, enabling one to lose weight. What I am most known and recognized for in the industry, and have recently been awarded a patent for, is taking an exercise that was considered anaerobic and being able to perform it for long periods or repetitions, giving the user (you) the advantage of both losing mass and toning at the same time *without* adding bulk but rather burning more fat during the time that you're exercising. This can be achieved by moving an object such as your own body weight and adding repetitions, building up to at least 50, rather than adding or increasing the weight and performing the traditional 8–12 repetitions for each exercise.

For example, if you typically use 10-pound dumbbells to perform a series of exercises such as triceps kick-backs and curls and perform three

Escape Route #43: The better shape you're in, the less oxygen you use, because you possess a greater margin of reserve and are capable of continuing on a high performance level for a longer period of time without distress to your body.

sets of 12 repetitions for each exercise, the total amount of weight moved during this routine equals 10 (pounds) × 12 (repetitions) × 3 (sets) = 360 pounds. For most people who are overweight and trying to lose mass and inches, even only 10 pounds can still be too much weight. They will bulk up because putting resistance or tension to more fat in any region of your body will only push the fat out farther due to the increased amount of muscle they add to that particular region. Thus they are building muscle faster than the rate at which they are burning fat or calories. Now, take a look at this workout scenario (which is completely outlined and illustrated in each of the weight-loss chapters): You use a two to four-pound Aerobic Toning bar and do 50 repetitions for those same two exercises, tricep kick-backs and curls, and perform three sets for each exercise, which equals four (pounds) × 50 (repetitions) × 3 (sets) = 600 pounds. As you can see, it is nearly twice the amount of weight pushed or moved using a *lighter* weight, but more important, because it is a lighter weight, for the purposes of losing mass you have extended the time (duration) of performing each exercise (burning more calories), building more muscle endurance (critical for elongating your muscles) and building more aerobic *and* anaerobic capacity, plus the cumulative weight you moved is nearly twice the amount and, most important, will trim your arms rather than bulking them up. This technique is the most effective for toning and losing mass and would not work for an individual who is trying to *gain* mass in any part or region of his/her body, but for all of you who are trying to *lose* mass, size, and weight, it is the only way to achieve your desired look.

As you become more fit, this same principle applies to each and every exercise you perform for both your upper and lower body as you try to shed weight and mass.

PHASE IV: COOLDOWN

After your workload, you must cool down by exercising at a gradually diminishing intensity. This prevents excessive pooling of the blood and muscle soreness, and it also protects the heart. Light aerobic movements such as walking or hiking at an easy pace for 2–3 minutes are the best ways to cool down.

Intensity and Target Heart Rate

Remember, just because you are exercising doesn't mean you will lose weight and/or change your body for the better. Aside from exercising in a manner that addresses all five components of fitness, following the four phases of a workout each and every time you work out, you now need to make sure you are exercising with enough intensity (how hard you are actually working while exercising). There are a number of ways to measure the proper intensity at which you should be exercising, and in my opinion, intensity is the second most important determining factor after frequency (the number of days you exercise) for achieving and maintaining weight loss. For first-time exercisers or beginners, it is also the most difficult thing to gauge. What's important to know about intensity in relation to weight loss is that you cannot lose weight on a continuous basis and possess a fit and toned body *without* increasing your level of fitness and you cannot vastly increase your level of fitness *without* increasing the intensity at which you are working out.

The reason that you need to keep increasing intensity (of which there are a number of ways) is because after you begin to exercise and increase your current level of fitness or lose weight by exercising, the physical demands on your system are not the same day 1 as they will be, say, on day 60. This is a perfect example of "plateauing," a term commonly used and heard throughout both the general population and fitness industry and one that is also completely misunderstood. It is not necessarily the *type* of exercise you need to change but the way you perform that particular exercise, with the proper intensity to determine your outcome. For instance, if you choose walking, jogging, biking, or jumping rope as your main aerobic component for your workouts, are you now supposed to *stop* performing these types of exercise because you have stopped losing weight or are not increasing your fitness level in these areas? Based on that theory, marathon runners, swimmers, cross-country skiers, and, for that matter, every single world-class athlete would suddenly *stop* their mode (type) of exercise and train performing other exercises, such as weight lifting, sprinting, or yoga. And what happens when these types of exercises are no longer effective? There's only so many exercises we can perform; it's not as if we have the time to perform thousands of exercises. I think you get my point. I can't remember for the life of me when a prizefighter or boxer substituted karate for boxing to prepare for a world championship match, can you? Most people plateau because they are not working hard enough during the time that they are performing their exercise(s).

For example, if you started out walking at three miles per hour for 30 minutes, the effect on your cardio system and the energy used (calories burned) would lessen over time as you became better conditioned. This is where your heart rate comes into play and is a *major* factor in both weight loss and increasing your current level of fitness. Your heart rate is an indication of how hard (intensity) you are working, so if you are 50

Escape Route #44: The heavier you are, the more calories you burn, and because your body is not used to exercising, *anything* you do fitness-wise creates an immediate caloric deficit in your favor; thus *initially* you will lose weight. Whether you keep up that weight loss, though, is determined by how consistent you are with your exercise regimen *coupled* with intensifying your workouts by small increments.

years old and take your heart rate on day 1 and it gets up to, let's say, 80 percent of your maximum heart rate (see heart rate section later in this chapter), your heart is beating an average of 136 beats per minute (BPM) to complete your 30-minute walk at three miles per hour. With frequency (number of times you walk per week), your heart rate will become lower if you don't change your speed and time (duration). Sixty days later, for that same 30-minute walk at three miles per hour, your heart rate is now 102 BPM, which represents only 60 percent of your maximum heart rate. It now takes less work for you to move your body and complete your walk, resulting in *fewer* calories being burned. You are now working more than 20 percent less each and every time you walk. Translation: you must now ingest 20 percent fewer calories in order to keep losing weight, which is highly unlikely. That's why people who only walk or choose one other type of exercise for weight loss initially lose weight but over time stop losing weight, because they are not exercising intensely enough to burn the same amount of calories as they did when they had begun.

There are a number of ways, though, that you can increase your intensity, ensuring that you'll keep burning calories while performing your walk: (1) you can extend the time (duration) you walk, (2) you can increase your speed, (3) you can increase your workload by adding hills, (4) you can walk with hand weights or a backpack, or (5) you can combine any two or all of these techniques together. Sounds simple, doesn't it? However, you must take into consideration a number of factors *before* you choose one or more techniques to increase your intensity, such as your medical and orthopedic background (perhaps you are on medication that affects your heart rate or have bad knees or a bad back), your goals (weight loss rather than toning or adding muscle mass), your lifestyle (does it allow for more time to be devoted to exercise?), and your current level of exercise.

When you extend the time of your workout, the shock to your heart, muscles, and system will be less than the other choices. Adding resistance (hills) will shoot your heart rate up quickly and possibly add mass (when overweight). Adding hand weights or a backpack will also shoot the heart rate up as well as put additional stress on your joints, especially your elbows and knees, and back. If your orthopedic background is not of solid foundation, then you need to switch your type (mode) of exercise, and your best choice would be a recumbent stationary bike, because you can increase the speed (RPMs) and duration without killing your joints. It's also important to note that this principle applies to not only walking but *any* type of exercise you perform, whether it be walking, jogging, weight lifting, yoga, or any type of exercise class.

Escape Route # 45: For the purposes of weight loss, the safest and most effective choice is to extend the time (duration) that you are walking, coupled with small increases in speed.

Next, you'll learn how to calculate your heart rate and measure the intensity at which you are exercising.

(THR) Calculating Your Target Heart Rate Zone

The intensity of your workout—how hard you're working—can make or break your fitness program. The easiest way for you to measure intensity during a fitness session is by checking your heart rate, that is, the number of times your heart beats in a minute. As you get in better shape, heart rate and target heart rate zone (THR) will increase because you'll be able to work harder without straining your heart as much. The more fit you become, the stronger your heart becomes. Even as you move into your sixties, seventies, and eighties you can continue to strengthen your heart with consistent and proper exercise, though as you age your target heart rate decreases.

Your THR is defined as the heart rate recommended during all forms of exercise for your age and fitness level. When you're in your THR zone, it means you're exercising with the proper intensity. Exercising above your THR means you're exercising too vigorously; exercising below your THR means you're not exercising vigorously enough. How hard should you work during exercise? The answer depends on several factors, but the threshold needed to achieve health benefits is lower for those who are sedentary than for those who are very fit. Your age, primary risk factors for heart disease, high blood pressure, medications, family history of heart disease, and stress levels, among other factors, dictate where you should begin.

To determine your heart rate zone, follow these steps:

1. Subtract your age from 220. This number represents your maximum heart rate. For example, a 50-year-old woman has a maximum heart rate of 170 (220 − 50 = 170). Her heart should not exceed 170 beats per minute during any type of physical activity. There are few exceptions. For instance, professional or well-trained amateur athletes may exceed that intensity. But most of you should monitor your heart rate during exercise, in part to avoid overexerting yourself.

2. To calculate the low end of your zone, multiply your maximum heart rate by .60. For our 50-year-old woman, that would be 170 × .60 = 102. That means in order to gain some benefits from her regime, she must work hard enough for her heart to beat at least 102 times per minute.

3. Calculate the high end of your zone by multiplying your maximum heart rate by .75. Our 50-year-old woman's is 170 × .75 = 128. So a 50-year-old semifit

woman whose goal is to lose weight should be exercising just hard enough for the heart to beat between 102 and 128 beats per minute.

How will your heart react when you begin or intensify your exercise program? That depends on how fit you are. The risk of heart problems is higher for sedentary people than for those who are more active. If you're a very active person, your heart is used to being taxed, though that's not to say an active lifestyle can substitute for a fitness program.

Most people start out with a program that's either under or over their zone. And very few warm up or stretch prior to increasing the intensity (energy) level. Remember, your heart jumps faster with anaerobic exercises than with aerobic ones. So use your THR zone as a guideline, then monitor your heart rate during exercise (also see "Gauge the Intensity of Your Workout"), since your heart rate increases as you increase the intensity of your activity.

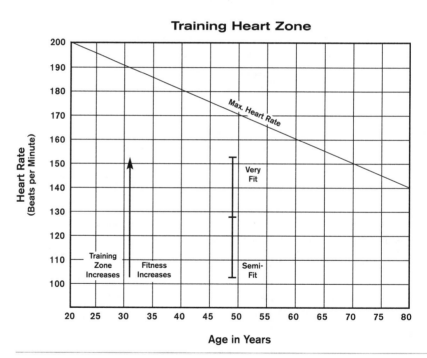

Training Heart Zone

EXAMPLES

A 50-year-old semifit individual
220 - 50 = 170 Maximum Heart Rate
Low End = .60 x 170 = 102 THR
High End = .75 x 170 = 128 THR

A 50-year-old very fit individual
Low End = .75 x 170 = 128 THR
High End = .90 x 170 = 153 THR

Gauge the Intensity of Your Workout

For beginners and/or those who are vastly overweight, when you embark on a new exercise program your heart rate should linger in the low end of your heart rate zone. **I strongly recommend that anyone over 35 years of age get a stress test done prior to engaging in any exercise or activity that causes his/her heart rate to go from a standing pulse (resting heart rate) to 75 percent of his/her maximal heart rate.**

Checking Your Heart Rate During Exercise

It's important to know your target zone before you begin exercising. (If you haven't done so already, see page 61 on how to do it.)

To monitor your heart rate during your workout:

- Slowly stop whatever you're doing and within three seconds locate your pulse at your neck, wrist, or temple with the tips of your index and middle fingers. Don't use your thumb, which has a pulse of its own. If taking your pulse on your chest, place the heel of your right hand over your heart.

- Use a clock with a second hand to count the number of beats for six seconds.

- Multiply that number by 10 to calculate your heart rate. That number represents how many times your heart is beating per minute during that particular exercise. If you're not in your zone, adjust your intensity level by either raising or lowering the intensity.

Take your pulse every 5 to 10 minutes during your workout. With practice you won't have to check your pulse so often. You'll simply feel and know how hard you're working. If you experience shortness of breath, find that you're not able to talk comfortably during aerobic exercise, or are feeling dizzy or nauseous, stop exercising immediately, place a wet, cool towel on your head, and lie down on your back, feet level with your head.

For beginners, it's more important to increase the time (duration) you spend exercising versus your intensity. Begin with low-intensity exercises, such as riding a stationary bike with light resistance or walking slowly on a treadmill. Remember that the more risk factors you have, the more critical it is for you to exercise closer to the low end or even under the low end of your zone. Your zone is only a range and a guide to follow. If you are exercising and find that you're huffing and puffing heavily, check your pulse. Even if you are still under your zone, decrease the intensity level immediately. And although you're under your prescribed zone, you are still getting benefits from the exercise. With time, you will be able to exercise comfortably within your zone and you'll even have to increase your intensity, so don't get discouraged.

Use your heart rate to monitor progress. I highly recommend heart-rate monitors for people with a heart complication. You strap this nifty device around your chest and it provides continuous feedback on how hard your heart is working. Heart monitors make it easy see to see if you are about to go above or below your zone, so you can adjust the intensity of your exertion conditions. While I've worked with countless people with heart conditions, each person's heart reacts differently to exercise, so if you are under a doctor's care regarding your heart, check with him/her to learn how to safely monitor your heart rate while performing any type of activity or exercise.

Remaining in your zone during your workout is important but doesn't necessarily mean you are becoming more fit or that your body will change in the areas that you expect it to. Many people who come to me for help exercise consistently within their target zones but do the wrong type of exercise for their goals, especially weight loss. For example, if you are overweight and happen to carry even more weight down below and are using step classes as your primary means of exercise, you'll never change your body to your desired level of satisfaction. Sure, you'll become a little more fit, but if you can become more fit, lose weight, and mold your body to your ideal at the same time, why not?

Ratings of Perceived Exertion (RPE)

Another popular means of measuring intensity during exercise is the "perceived exertion" scale. Rather than using a formula, Borg's scale, also know as the Ratings of Perceived Exertion (RPE), was developed to allow exercisers to subjectively rate their feelings during exercise, taking into account personal fitness level, environmental conditions, and general fatigue. Currently, two RPE scales are widely used: the original, which rates exercise intensity on a scale of 6 to 20, and the revised scale, on which you can rate exertion from 0 to 10. I use the revised scale with my clients because the terminology is easier to understand, though both scales account for the increase in heart rate during exercise.

You don't have to be quick or good with numbers to use the Borg scale. While exercising, you simply ask yourself, "How hard am I exerting myself?" and assign a number value to your answer. The low end of the scale (0) means you're not exerting yourself at all. The high end of the scale (10) represents the point at which you could push yourself no harder. If you feel that you are at a 3, then based on your medical background and unique constraints (if any), you can pick up intensity or lower it. After rating your exertion, you may want to take your pulse. It should fall somewhere in the zone that you've chosen according to your goals. I highly recommend this scale for healthy individuals. For those who are vastly out-of-shape or need special medical attention, use a heart-rate monitor to ensure safety. Today you will find most treadmills, stationary bikes, steppers, ellipticals, or the like with built-in heart monitors.

RPE is very helpful not only as a guide for working out with the proper intensity but also as a tool to gauge how fit you are becoming performing the same exercise over time.

Revised Scale for Ratings of Perceived Exertion (RPE)

0	Nothing at all
0.5	Very, very weak
1	Very weak
2	Weak
3	Moderate
4	Somewhat strong
5	Strong
6	Underscore
7	Very Strong
8	Underscore
9	Underscore
10	Very, very strong, maximal

Taken from ACSM's *Guidelines for Exercise Testing and Prescription*, 5th ed. (1995).

Safeguarding Yourself

If you're out walking or hiking, what are you supposed to do immediately after spraining an ankle or straining your hamstring? A good way to remember what steps you should take to get yourself back to 100 percent is through this simple acronym—***PRICE.***

P: *PROTECT* your body and, more specifically, the body part that's injured from further injury. If you continue to exercise and aggravate the injured area when you get hurt, you're only asking for trouble.

The first and foremost rule for preventing further damage while performing any exercise or sport is that if a part of your body is hurting stop immediately. It doesn't make you less of a person to walk off the tennis or basketball court because you twisted your ankle.

> *Escape Route #46:*
> Ceasing exercise is the first phase in treating an athletic-related injury.

Following are common exercises and activities and the body parts they usually affect most:

- Basketball: ankles, knees, calves, head, eyes.

- Downhill skiing: knees ankles, back, head.

- Exercise/aerobic classes, step classes, stair climbers: knees, ankles, back, feet, shins, calves.

- Golf: back, forearms, upper arms, hips.

- Horseback riding: back, hips, knees, legs.

- Jumping rope: calves, back, knees if jumping on hard surface.

- Racquet sports: eyes, head, rear thighs, groin, calves, feet.

- Rowing: knees, back.

- Running/jogging: ankles, knees, back, heels, calves, feet, shins, hips, front and rear thighs.

- Softball: shoulders, ankles, knees.

- Tennis: calves, groin, thighs, hamstrings.

- Touch football: ankles, knees, calves, thighs, hamstrings, Achilles.

- Walking: back, knees.

- Weight lifting: neck, back, hips, feet, front and rear thighs, shoulders, chest.

- Yoga: strained and torn muscles throughout body.

Escape Route #47: Most injuries occur because of lack of proper warm-up and stretching beforehand or poor fitness levels.

If you are susceptible to certain injuries, please take extra precautions while playing any sport or engaging in any exercise.

The next phase in treating yourself for injury is **R**, for *REST. Rest* does not mean walking it off. You cannot and will not walk off an ankle sprain or muscle strain. Such an injury requires, among other things, immediate rest. Rest also means to rest until it is just about completely healed. Isn't it better to rest your calf a couple of days after injuring it, rather than risk pulling or tearing it and missing the next 6–12 weeks?

Next on the list is *I,* for *ICE.* Take a plastic bag, put 10–20 ice cubes in it, and tie it. Put it in another bag to prevent leakage. Then apply the bag directly to the injury with a five-inch Ace bandage so it does not fall off. Apply for stints of 20–40 minutes twice a day until all the swelling or major pain has subsided. If it takes you five days to heal, then apply ice for five days.

Next we have **C**, for *COMPRESSION*—not just compression with the ice but also after icing, making sure that the injury is sufficiently wrapped, with the right amount of pressure. Not too light and not too heavy. Compression allows the swelling to dissipate more quickly than just laying the ice bag on the injury. I cannot overemphasize the importance of icing and compression after an injury.

Finally, **E**, for *ELEVATE*. Make sure that while you are icing, sleeping, resting, watching TV, or reading, the body part that is injured the most is elevated. This allows the blood to flow smoothly to the injured area.

There is no substitution for the PRICE system. Do not ignore the fact that you're injured. Everybody gets a little bruise or bump or strains themselves at some time. And remember, the most important thing when you injure yourself is to ice the injured part and rest long enough for your injury to heal. If you are not sure what to do after getting hurt, ask a doctor who is familiar with your type of injury. Obviously, the best way to protect yourself against injury is to become fit before going out there and playing any sport that requires a reasonable level of fitness.

For instance, if you are going to take an exercise class or go out and play hoops, first weigh the benefits against the risks. Just because you used to be in great shape and dominated a particular sport 10 or more years ago, don't think your body will respond in the same way today, especially if you've not kept up with a conditioning program.

Another common mistake made by many who exercise is exercising out of their heart rate zone. Be especially careful in very hot or very cold climates, as the heart may not take the stress. Inexperience can get you into trouble as well. If you do not know where to position yourself on a tennis court when playing tennis doubles, don't be shocked when you have ball marks on the backs of your legs by the end of your tennis day.

The older you are, the more risk you have of skeletal injuries. And if you have a special medical condition make sure there is a medical facility nearby if you're engaging in any vigorous activity.

Muscle soreness, especially when beginning an exercise program, is quite common. If you cannot get out of bed the next day you definitely overdid it. But if you wake up and your body feels slightly sore, then you did just the right amount of exercise. In a week or two, this soreness will dissipate. If it does not, check with your doctor. Warming up, stretching, and cooling down help muscle soreness, as well as performing your exercises with proper form and alignment. Most people know when there is something wrong with their body. Listen to it. Nine out of ten times

Escape Route #48: Do not apply heat after any injury. If you are not sure what to do, ask your doctor or local pharmacist.

Escape Route #49: Stay away from exercises or sports that you know aggravate parts of your body where you are weak or have orthopedic problems.

you're right. **Do not ignore warning signals when exercising.** The pain will not go away if you ignore it; it will only get worse. On the other hand, if you turn your ankle, rest a day or so, but start getting back into your exercise regimen by biking, stretching, and performing any exercise that does not inflame the ankle. If you work out the rest of your body while injured, you will heal faster, because the body is sending signals to the injured area. In addition, atrophy will not set in as fast.

A common mistake made by many who exercise, especially first-timers, is not distinguishing muscle fatigue and discomfort from actual pain. Muscle fatigue is a general feeling of tiredness throughout the entire muscle that you've been exercising. The muscle may feel sore and/or tight. Pain, however, will be a more localized, intense sensation. If you're doing sit-ups and your stomach muscles feel tired and tight, you can keep going a little bit more. But if you get a sharp, stabbing pain after just one or two repetitions, stop and consult with a health professional. Confusing muscle fatigue with pain can lead to injury. It's a tough thing to distinguish, especially for those just starting out. If you're not sure how to perform a particular exercise, seek advice from someone knowledgeable within the fitness industry.

Which would you prefer—to not ask and get hurt or to ask, learn, and possibly never injure yourself? For some strange reason, most people are very shy about asking questions about exercise and they think it's embarrassing to ask. How can you expect to know about a particular field or industry if you are not schooled? You need to study and gain experience in any field of fitness to be an expert. It's no different from being a plumber, accountant, lawyer, or doctor. So, the next time you're hesitant to ask, throw away your ego and do it.

Proper footwear and clothing are also helpful in preventing injuries and overheating. Go out and spend some money on the right apparel. If your plumber showed up with carpenter tools, could he do an effective job? Wear clothes that breathe, preferably cotton. There are more sports shops and sneaker outlets today than one can count. Go in and ask the most knowledgeable person for advice. And when a couple of them from different stores agree with each other, then you can make the right purchase.

Escape Route #50: Do not ask your friends for advice on what you should do if you have injured yourself. When in doubt, ask a professional—be it exercise or, for that matter, any subject that you're not sure what steps are needed to take to ensure safety, proper form, and technique.

In Summary

Now that you know what to do in preparation for beginning your weight-loss regimen, here are some motivational and helpful tips to ensure that you don't forget anything in your quest to slim down. The most important thing to keep in mind while trying to lose weight is what your true goal is.

Try to keep in mind that from time to time you will get off track by either overeating and/or skipping your workouts. Remember, losing weight is a process, and if and when you get sidetracked, don't despair and lose confidence; dig down deep and get back on track by learning from your mistakes and focus all of your energy on eating smarter and exercising with the proper intensity and consistency. Also, no matter what happens, try not to let more than two days go by *without* performing at least 30–45 minutes of sustained aerobic exercise, because it is your insurance policy for helping you take and keep weight off. And if you do overeat now and then, again, get on that bike or treadmill and help whisk away those extra calories instead of "starving" yourself or "dieting."

Another important tip concerns when and how often to weigh yourself: ***Don't*** weigh yourself when you have had a bad day or two of eating or have not exercised during that time frame. ***Do*** weight yourself after you have had a good run of eating well and exercising consistently.

Some lifestyle experts and dieticians don't believe in weighing yourself at all, and if you are within, let's say, five pounds of your ideal weight and inches are more important than pounds, then I agree. But if you are overweight by more than ten pounds, it is *very* important to weigh yourself for a few reasons: (1) it holds you accountable for your behavior and actions, (2) it helps you analyze what adjustments you need to make in adjusting either your eating or exercise plan or both, and (3) based on the number on the scale (whether you've lost weight, remained the same weight, or gained weight), you can look back at your behavior during this time frame and make any necessary changes to your weight-loss plan.

Try to weigh yourself once a week on the same day and at the same time. Typically, we weigh less in the morning than the evening because we have not consumed a whole day of calories yet, especially if we exercised the evening before.

Also, weigh yourself on the same scale each and every time, because not all scales are the same and if your scale is plus or minus a pound or two compared to, let's say, your doctor's scale, it doesn't matter, because if your scale moves upward or downward when you do weigh yourself *your* scale is still a true measure of your current weight gain or loss. And if your scale is off let's say by two pounds and according to your scale you are now five pounds lighter after a week or two of eating well and exercising consistently, by getting on a different scale that registers you as only three pounds lighter you will become very disappointed and might become discouraged. The reality of the situation is that you *have* lost five

Escape Route #51: Instead of being obsessed with losing weight, channel your energy and efforts and become obsessed with creating a clear path to eating sensibly six out of seven days and exercising five days per week, week after week. Because if you are able to do this, with time you will reach your goal. You'll not only lose weight, but equally important, you'll keep it off and remain fit for the rest of your life.

pounds because *your* scale indicates so. If you are on medication or hormone replacements or have any other special medical needs, there may be times when the scale is not moving in a downward direction *despite* the fact that you are eating well and exercising like a fiend. Again, don't despair, make an appointment with your doctor or health care professional, and ask him/her if this is normal and, if so, can he/she possibly prescribe a different medication that will not compromise your health yet will also not hinder you as much in achieving consistent weight loss. If this is not possible, don't worry, because even though it might take longer for your body to lose weight, with time your metabolism will adjust and eventually speed up, but *only* through exercise, not by cutting caloric intake alone.

And last, aside from eating sensibly and exercising consistently, start becoming more active. Pick an activity or sport that you enjoy and slowly get into it. Remember your Habit Atlas? (Chapter 1) Each and every thing you do affects weight loss and adds up in your favor, just as doing very little in the way of being active counts against you. Plus, if your everyday diet (total of calories you consume daily) remains the same for this time frame, because you are more active you will create an easy deficit in your favor and thus it will be reflected on the scale when you do your weekly weigh-in.

Want to Be More Active?

To help you make smart choices when choosing an activity or exercise, I have put together a chart of some common activities/exercises and the amount of calories that you would burn during a half hour of continuous movement. Keep in mind that this is an average only; some people will burn more calories during this time frame and some individuals will burn fewer calories, depending upon how intensely or vigorously they are moving.

Activities/Exercise Average Calories Burned During 30 Minutes	140– 160 lbs.	160– 180 lbs.	180– 200 lbs.	200– 220 lbs.	220– 240 lbs.
Jumping rope @135 turns a minute	570	660	720	780	840
Aerobics (traditional)	276	313	362	392	430
Basketball	282	319	358	397	436
Bowling	45	53	62	70	79
Cleaning the attic or garage (no stairs)	65	75	85	95	105
Cycling	205	232	259	286	313
Gardening: Planting	156	168	179	192	205
Gardening: Digging	260	275	290	305	320
Gardening: Weeding	170	190	210	230	250
Golf (carry clubs)	174	198	222	246	270
Golf (power cart)	79	90	102	114	126
Hiking	168	190	213	237	261
Jogging (5.0–6.0 mph)	348	394	439	484	529
Making beds	102	112	122	132	142
Moving furniture	290	302	314	326	338
Mowing the lawn	200	220	240	260	280
Running (6.0+ mph)	424	481	538	595	652
Reading	42	48	54	60	66
Scrubbing the kitchen floor with mop	95	115	130	145	160
Skating (ice and roller)	222	250	277	304	331
Skiing (cross-country)	282	319	357	393	429
Skiing (downhill and water)	213	241	268	295	322
Swimming (moderate pace)	289	328	367	406	445
Tennis	222	252	280	307	334
Vacuuming	90	98	106	114	122
Walking (moderate pace) (3.0–4.2 mph)	244	276	306	336	366
Washing windows	90	100	110	120	130
Weight training	244	277	310	343	376

*Sources include: ACSM, ACE, AFAA, American Heart Association, and CookingLight.com.

IT DOESN'T MATTER WHAT PLAN

OF ACTION YOU CHOOSE TO

LOSE WEIGHT AS LONG AS THE

PLAN YOU'VE CHOSEN IS

HEALTHY AND ONE THAT YOU

CAN ADHERE TO WITHOUT

DEVIATING!

CHAPTER FOUR

Choosing the Right Formula for Success

What You "Think" You're Willing to Do Versus What You're Actually Going to Do

During the last twenty years of designing lifestyle and fitness programs, I always sat down and listened to what my clients had to say regarding their medical and orthopedic background, lifestyle, and current commitment level. By "commitment level" I mean, based on what they need to accomplish, whether it's weight loss, improvement of their overall health, or an increase of their fitness level, their willingness to do what's necessary in order to realize their sought-after wishes. I often find that people's bark is much bigger than their actual bite. For example, I cannot tell you how many times an individual who hasn't worked out a day in his/her life other than walking to and from his/her refrigerator strolls in and tells me how he/she is "willing to do whatever it takes" to lose weight and that he/she has "tried everything" out there, but it hasn't worked. Then he/she proceeds to tell me that he/she will exercise seven days a week and swears that he/she will follow our nutritionist's advice, with no deviations. Now don't get me wrong, I love this individual's enthusiasm and feel quite flattered and fortunate that he/she has chosen my firm to help get him/her to his/her desired weight-loss and fitness goals, but . . .

The first thing I do after listening to them is explain that they haven't tried "everything" in their quest for weight loss. Then I proceed to ask them if they have ever performed a full-body exercise regimen five days per week coupled with following an eating plan that *does not* involve any extreme dieting for 90 days? To date, I have yet to meet a person who has

Escape Route #52:
Sometimes what people "think" they're going to do and what they're "actually" going to do do not match up.

answered "yes" to this question. Being the curious lad that I am, of course I ask them, "Why not?" And most of them state that no one ever taught them a process by which they could eat real food without giving up carbs or proteins, et cetera, and according to their doctor, the only exercise that was expected of them was walking or a mild exercise class.

So after hearing them explain to me their war stories, being the rational person I am, I then ask them if they have never exercised *properly* with any kind of consistency **prior** to coming in to Exude, what makes them think that they can possibly work out seven days a week as they boldly told me when we started our conversation just a few minutes ago? It's important to note here that I ask these questions not to embarrass them or make them feel uncomfortable but rather to get them to take a step back and let them realize that they are setting themselves up for a big disappointment and, more important, failure before they even begin. Not because they don't have the ability, I explain, but because of the process or plan that they have chosen in order to reach their weight-loss goals. And now the most important question I ask is: "Susan [Bob], which are you more apt to do, in other words, what do you have more of a problem sticking to, dieting or exercise?" And it doesn't matter what the reason is that he/she feels an affinity for either one. "What's important," I explain, "is being honest with yourself, because your answer **dictates** the plan and process that we will design for you. Without this information, even with the best of intentions, your odds of sticking to *any* weight-loss program are minimal at best. If you loathe exercise as most people do, just because I prescribe that you work out six days a week is hardly insurance that you'll actually do it week in and week out. And how do I know that? Because I already asked you if you have ever exercised with that kind of regularity during the last forty-five years of being on this earth and you told me no. Developing the habits and skills to eat sensibly and exercise properly and consistently takes time. It is unrealistic to think that after spending an hour with me you are now emancipated and magically possess the discipline, knowledge, and motivation to eat properly and work out consistently for the rest of your life. If that were the case, I'd be the pope and all I would need to do is travel the world and just bless people and their problems would be solved, and I hardly think that I am that saintly."

The main reason, by the way, that most people loathe exercise is because they have never really exercised in a manner that gave them visible results. As you now have read and learned from my previous chapters, walking on a treadmill or taking an exercise class is **not** fitness but rather a form of exercise, and you also now know that exercise and fitness are not one and the same. Aside from confusion as to how to eat, what to eat, and when and how often to exercise, mixed in with knowing how to exercise efficiently in order to burn enough calories, nine out of ten people don't truly understand that weight loss and fitting proper and consistent exercise into their everyday lives require a game plan according to their lifestyle and, more important, likes and dislikes toward dieting (in regard to eating less only) versus exercise. In other words, each person has a distinct personality and, based on his/her history from childhood, is more apt to find it easier to cut calories rather than exercise four, five, or six days per week. Or some people are willing to exercise those six days per week yet are not comfortable "dieting." And then there are those who are willing and don't find it taxing to their system to exercise four or five days per week and make small changes in their caloric intake (eat less).

My favorite, and quite effective, tip for motivating you to lose weight and go down in dress, suit, or pant size is to give away all of your clothing that no longer can be saved by having it altered. Too often, people keep these clothes lying around in their closet as a "safety" net in case they put the weight back on, as they have quite often done in the past. Giving away this clothing makes people think twice about giving up, because most people don't have thousands of dollars lying around or, better yet, are too embarrassed to go out and shop for a whole new wardrobe.

And think of the time you'll save by just popping into any store and being able to choose what you want to wear versus what you have to or need to purchase in order to not turn and ask your friend, "Do I look fat in this?"

The problem is, you are going to look fat in anything you buy if *you are fat,* the only difference being, of course, that in some outfits you look even more overweight and others you don't look as overweight. But believe me, you still look overweight. Whether you realize or believe or accept the fact, it's obvious that you care about what others think about your appearance; otherwise, you would never ask your friend or second-guess yourself when you do try on clothing. And there's nothing wrong with that. If you're overweight and are happy with the way you look naked and are comfortable with that, then OK. But, to date, I have never met an overweight individual who has said to me or, more important, to him/herself that he/she feels good and didn't wish he/she were in better shape or, at the very least, slimmer.

That's why I laugh (and cringe) when I read or hear an interview with women and men in Hollywood who state emphatically that they have

Escape Route #53:
Wouldn't it be wonderful to finally go shopping for clothing that compliments your body rather than search for clothing that "hides" or covers up your body? There's a big difference, you know, between the two.

"tried everything," but it hasn't worked, and now they have resigned themselves in their minds to this being the way they are going to look for the rest of their career (it will be short and with very few lead roles, I assure you) and if we (the public) don't like it, then too bad. Again, they have not tried everything; they have only tried extreme ways of trying to lose weight and have failed because of the path they chose. Based on that theory, everyone including myself, who eats sensibly (most of the time, anyway) and exercises regularly and properly should be blimps, right? This sends a *wrong* message to all viewers or listeners across America and for that matter worldwide, that it's OK to look, feel, and function this way. Think real hard and tell me how many A-list actors and actresses are vastly overweight today? Not many, huh? Also along these lines, how about the number of A-list hosts of television shows, news shows, and the like? Again, not a high number. Do you know why? Because the networks know that it is bad for ratings. In their minds, no one wants to look at a vastly overweight person on TV because it's bad for their image and gives the impression that he/she doesn't care about how he/she takes care of or presents him/herself or looks to his/her viewers. Remember, I am just the messenger; don't shoot me. I want you to take your anger and energy and focus on becoming the best that *you* can become, and I promise that with time your entire life will improve as you start gravitating toward your weight-loss goals. The *key* is to be honest with yourself, make the correct decisions, and stick to that game plan without deviating.

Three Effective Options for Losing Weight

Here I have outlined and described *three* distinctly unique methods for shedding weight that mimic and match up to what an individual will actually stick to as he/she begins his/her journey toward weight loss. There are only three ways to safely, effectively, and efficiently achieve and maintain weight loss through proper eating and exercise. A number of factors affect that choice and influence your decision, most of which have to do with your life during and since childhood, such as how active you were, the sports you may or may not have participated in, dieting as a teen, eating and drinking habits, and whether you have been exercising, and, if so, how long you've been working out. So, before you choose your plan of action, take a look at all three options and choose the one that best matches and copies your personality. You may find in reading about these three different styles that you possess one, a few, or all of these traits. Please note that I am merely presenting the facts and observations I made based on the many thousands of individuals I have met with and consulted with over the years from which these characteristics and patterns were drawn and not in any way judging your behavior. I am only concerned with educating and motivating you to choose the right game plan based on your likes and dislikes concerning diet and exercise so that you are able to reach all of your weight-loss and fitness goals by looking at the factors that *today* you can control. It's also important to note here that you *cannot* make up your own set of laws or mix and match wherever you desire when choosing your game plan. For instance, you can't choose to make no dietary changes whatsoever yet also refuse to exercise and expect to be successful at weight loss. Conversely, you also cannot choose to only "diet" without some ingredient of exercise present, either.

Keep in mind that it is your current viewpoints, behavior in the past, and habits, both good and bad, that dictate your initial approach. All three of the options I provide can be effective, but you want to increase your chances of success and lower your risk of failure by making small adjustments and changes, eliminating or at least minimizing extreme behavior, and working toward achieving weight loss by slowly gravitating toward creating a better balance between consistent exercise and eating sensibly. The method you choose should reflect the behavior, attitude, and approach toward weight loss that you feel most comfortable and familiar with currently. Everyone wants to better themselves, and deep down we all know that we should exercise consistently and eat sensibly without "dieting." Losing weight is not very different from trying to achieve any other task or goal or overcome a dilemma or hurdle in our lives. There is nothing wrong with being overweight other than not trying to better yourself just as you aspire to be better as a parent or in your job or any other endeavor you seek to master. And sometimes it takes experimenting and fine-tuning, even failing, before we realize that we need to take a step back and analyze the process that we've chosen, which may need to be tweaked and improved upon.

The most important thing you need to know about weight loss is that if you *truly* give 100 percent, you can only succeed.

And don't get me wrong; achieving weight loss is no walk in the park; it's difficult but hardly impossible. You need to put yourself completely in my hands and guidance even if you don't "like" what guidance I give you, because one thing is for sure—your way is not working and if you can put your ego aside and be open-minded, I promise you'll get to the promised land. It might be rocky, but hey, nothing good in life, as you well know, is easy. You have to earn the right to look and feel great;

> *Escape Route #54:* How often did you give 100 percent and failed? I bet it happened far less often than you failed and did not give that same effort.

you're not entitled to be fit and trim just because you want to be. The old adage "you get what you put into it" holds true even with weight loss. Although plausibly simple, eating sensibly and exercising properly and consistently is complex, not the process itself but creating a clear path with your unique lifestyle, habits, prejudices, and likes and dislikes that perhaps get in the way, cloud the issue, and prevent you from making smart choices. My goal is to make you aware of these pitfalls and experiences so that you'll learn from your mistakes, because all that really matters, is when you wipe away all the fluff, the bottom line and determining factor in whether you lose weight is based solely on the total amount of calories that remain or leave your body on a consistent basis.

All of the three approaches featured here are the only means that you, me, or your neighbor or spouse has either tried in the past or is currently using. And all of them have pros and cons, and each and every method can be improved upon. Your task is to pick the one that you will stick to based upon your likes and dislikes in relation to food and exercise. Try to make small adjustments by applying some or all of the tips. By doing so, you will vastly improve your odds and chances for permanent weight loss. There is more than just one way to get to your desired weight, just as there is more than one way to solve any other dilemma or problem. Your *problem* is not that you're overweight per se; it has more to do with the *route* you choose to solve your dilemma.

Here are your options.

Option #1, Limited Approach—Weight Loss Through Restriction of Calories

BACKGROUND AND PERSPECTIVE ON DIET AND EXERCISE

Put simply, for you the thought of regular exercise is about as appealing as the thought of baby-sitting a family of crocodiles. Dieting or cutting calories is much easier for you to stick to with regularity and it isn't as taxing to you physiologically as well as psychologically as working out is. You fight and have been resistant to fitness for years. You're the type that never liked gym class as a child, and you either cut gym class or hid in the corner of the gymnasium, avoiding it like the plague because either you weren't blessed with the same athletic ability as your peers or no one ever took the time to teach you the skills necessary to play sports and thus you never had confidence that you could actually be good at sports. When sides were chosen for a sport such as softball, you were the kid they stuck in short centerfield, batting last, thus assuring that you could do no damage to your team. You always felt enormous pressure and perhaps were even snickered at by your classmates each and every time you attempted to do anything that involved physical fitness. You might have also been an underweight, skinny, or weak child or overweight as a child and couldn't keep up and compete physically with your counterparts. If you were overweight since a teenager, you have tried a number of "diets" that are extreme in nature and hope for a magical pill or shortcut out there somewhere that's bound to work, as long as you don't have to sweat. You get easily discouraged when trying a new diet that hasn't worked and have resolved in your mind and accepted the fact that the reason you cannot win at weight loss is either "genetic" or something about you and you alone. In short, you have very little confidence that you'll ever be fit and trim.

You typically are well read, more so than the average person, and consider yourself intellectually smarter than most people because, quite simply, you are less active, have less active-type hobbies, and have spent most of your time or life focusing on things such as reading, which require very little physical activity. You eat out of boredom and/or depression and initially do well with "diets" but cannot sustain them for long periods of time. You have lost more pounds over the years of dieting than your current weight but always put them back on, and quite often the amount you put back on is more than you have lost. You could write a book on dieting; you just cannot write a book on how to be successful at dieting. You may have even tried diet or overweight centers, farms, or spas, and while they were somewhat successful, three or four months later as you tried to maintain that weight loss you always ended up putting it back on. You are the classic yo-yo dieter or perhaps have even given up at this time attempting any type of eating plan or weight-loss program.

Or you could be one of these fortunate-type people who have been "naturally" thin almost their entire childhood and adult life and who were very disciplined with their eating. You never had to "diet," but you were careful with not overeating and you were always conscious of the calories you were consuming because you didn't exercise and, in your mind, never had to because you were never overweight and you looked at exercise as a chore and only something that heavy or overweight people need to do to shed weight, but not you. Over the years, though, as you focused on your career and/or family, you found that you have started putting on the pounds, especially around your midsection, and now you are starting to panic a bit. Now you're forced to do something, and since you have avoided exercise like the plague nearly your entire life, you would rather diet than begin exercising, even though you know you should start working out despite your prejudices.

It is unrealistic to think that you're going to start exercising four or five days a week right out of the box, especially since you have never done so in your entire life. Besides, the thought of "dieting" or cutting calories is much more familiar to you, and given the choice between dieting and exercise, you know that you would be more likely to follow the former rather than the latter. What I cannot understand for the life of me yet is how you have the willpower to diet and deprive yourself like you do, which requires much more focus and determination than exercising a few days a week for an hour each clip. It's mind-boggling to me, and as of the time during which I am writing this book, what drives anyone to choose this path is one of the very few things I've yet to uncover.

Like I often say, "it is what it is," so here are some things that you need to be aware of as you attempt to lose weight while choosing this method.

If you're going to primarily rely on cutting calories to lose weight, with only a "sprinkle" of exercise thrown in, your formula for success does not leave you a lot of leeway for error. You are only required to exercise two times a week for forty-five minutes or so, combined with following a strict eating plan. The downside to choosing this alternative is that if and when you go off course with your eating here and there, since you are only working out twice a week your only option for losing the extra weight that you gained because of not eating perfectly is to further cut your calories to make up for the excess calories that you consumed.

Your other option, of course, is to exercise more frequently, but that's not happening; otherwise you would not have chosen to lose weight by this means, would you? This method of severely cutting caloric intake also slows down your MBR, and if and when you lose the weight and are happy with what the scale indicates, the minute you start going back to eating "normally," which automatically means ingesting more calories, you will only put that weight back on and quite possibly even more weight than you had worked so diligently to take off. Remember, no deviations if you choose this means for losing weight. It will work, but you have to be resigned to the fact that for your *entire* life in order to maintain this weight loss you will never be able to enjoy the finer things that life has to offer. In other words, you cannot decide that one day you're fed up with "dieting" and no longer are willing to deprive yourself like you have been doing without facing the consequence, and that is quite a simple fact: you will gain weight. If you have the willpower to follow this plan and you think that you have it in you for the long haul (lifetime), then good luck, my friend, and by the way, I want to meet you, because in over 20 years of being in this industry I have never met an individual who has mastered this method for years on end.

TIPS TO CREATE A BETTER BALANCE

The process for creating a better balance between eating sensibly and incorporating more and regular exercise into your daily life has to be done so that it isn't too shocking to your lifestyle. Try some of the following:

- Pick and choose an active hobby such as gardening, bird-watching/walking, hiking, cross-country skiing, downhill skiing, running minimarathons, doubles tennis, golf, et cetera. By doing so, you will be more apt to exercise so that you can enjoy your favorite activity or sport, because you will possess more confidence in your physical abilities as well as increase your fitness level. In other words, instead of viewing your fitness sessions as torturous or boring you can now look at them as helping you get more out of your hobby.

- Try to pick more active friends and/or associates. By doing so, when you get together socially your chances are greater of doing something active than when you are hanging out with some of your not-so-active couch potato friends.

- If you feel self-conscious and are uncomfortable exercising among your peers or total strangers, invest in some home fitness equipment so that you ensure that you will be exercising. If you are comfortable exercising around others, join a health club or gym and try to form a relationship with someone who exercises at the same time as you and develop a support system with him/her.

- On weekends, when you have more time to work out, add more time to your workouts, and make sure that you exercise each Saturday and Sunday. The more often you work out the faster you'll lose weight, and eventually you will be more apt to exercise with more frequency during the workweek.

- Make realistic goals and when you hit certain weight-loss benchmarks reward yourself with such things as a massage or a new pair of shoes—in short, make yourself *earn* them.

- If and when you go off course and overindulge with your eating or imbibing, instead of "starving" yourself for two or three days to make up for those extra calories, work out an extra day or two that week. By doing so, you will become less dependent on dieting and create a more balanced approach to weight loss.

- Try to slowly increase your caloric intake with healthy food on the days that you are working out. As long as your total calories consumed those particular days do not exceed your allowed caloric intake, you will continue to lose weight and soon realize that you can have a little more leeway with your diet without having to worry about gaining weight.

In summary, make sure that you stick to your strict eating guidelines based upon your weight-loss category outlined in part 2. Try to keep in mind that the less you work out and exercise, the more careful and diligent you need to be with your eating plan.

To be successful in using this approach to weight loss, you need to work out a minimum of two times per week, with your ultimate goal to be increasing your exercise frequency to four times per week, thus ensuring that you'll never have to "diet" another day for the rest of your life.

Option #3, Dynamic Approach—Weight Loss Through Excessive Activity

BACKGROUND AND PERSPECTIVE ON DIET AND EXERCISE

Just as it's unrealistic to expect a nonexerciser to suddenly begin exercising with great frequency, it is equally unrealistic to think that you can follow a very restrictive diet right from the start. You're the type that lives to eat versus eats to live. You would rather work out seven days a week than even think about dieting. That's why you exercise so much, because you use it as a balancing of the scales. For example, you know you're going out to eat a fine dinner or have a sit-down home-cooked meal with all the trimmings—hence, you exercise like a fiend.

You also fear gaining weight, and that's a great motivating factor to keep you moving at all times. From childhood, you were either a tomboy or a jock and played organized sports or excelled in individual sports. You ate and drank as much as you wanted and countered it with moving as much as you could. Today, because you are older and don't have as much time to devote to exercise, you may have turned into a weekend warrior, getting most of your workouts done during weekends. You have been slowly putting on weight because you refuse to ease up on your eating despite the fact that you are only half as active as you used to be. You also may think that you're still twenty-one years old and, at forty, you can still physically do what you were able to do some twenty years ago.

You fear getting old and still may even participate in organized sports such as basketball, hockey, rugby, or football with your buddies, and then afterward, of course, you hit the bar, throw a few drinks down, and then go home and eat a full dinner. Growing up, when you were told to eat everything on your plate you were one of the few to actually listen and do so. That habit formed way back then is still ingrained into your soul, and to this day you eat whatever is presented to you on your plate even if you feel full. As a youth, you were stocky or even overweight, yet because of your athleticism and/or determination you could somewhat keep up with your counterparts physically. As a young adult, either you shed some weight and were fortunate enough to play college sports or club sports or you tried to control your weight strictly through exercise. You love working out, pushing yourself to the max, and even exercising through pain. From running or lifting weights to taking exercise classes, nothing is too big to conquer from a fitness standpoint. You may have tinkered with a diet or two in the past but found that you had low energy and/or were miserable while attempting to do so. You get frustrated when you cannot work out because you know that you won't be able to enjoy your next meal as much and inevitably will have to work out even harder the next time you can exercise, to make up for the weight gain during your dormant period. When I design weight-loss programs for this extreme-type behavior, I always ask these people why they work out so often. Some people respond by telling me they truly enjoy exercising every day and others state that they like to eat, so in order to not gain weight it is necessary in their minds to work out daily.

But if I delve deeper as to the actual reason those who told me they enjoy exercise do it so excessively and inquire about their eating and drinking habits, I notice that their eating and drinking habits are no different from those of the people who explained to me that they exercise so often because of their eating habits. "Don't get me wrong," I explain. "I'm sure you do enjoy exercising so often, but even professional athletes don't work out seven days a week and it would do you and your body a great service if you cut down to at least six or even five days per week."

It is just as difficult to get someone to *lower* his/her frequency (days per week) of exercise as it is to get someone to *increase* his/her frequency. They are just on different ends of the spectrum. Both exhibit extreme behavior, but what motivates them to choose their path is not important. What is important is to make you aware of your behavior and habits and the pros and cons of your decisions so that you can make small adjustments toward altering your extreme behavior and find a better balance, thus increasing your odds of losing weight and maintaining that weight loss for the long haul without the pressure of exercising daily.

YOUR FITNESS AND DIET GAME PLAN

It's important to point out here that even though you are moving or exercising with such frequency the *type* of exercise you perform is still critical to your success or failure in weight loss. Often people who are so active or exercise so much are not aware that sure, they're moving, but it is not the correct form of exercise to counter the total amount of food consumed that particular day or week. Make sure you are performing sustained (at least 30 minutes) intense aerobic activity six times per week in addition to all of your other fitness and active endeavors. It's the aerobic exercise that will help you lose that mass and weight, not the anaerobic. Also, choose more aerobic-type activities such as hiking, jogging, basketball, volleyball, singles tennis, biking, et cetera. Golf, walking the course, is not purely aerobic because you are only walking a few hundred yards, stopping, and hitting your ball, and waiting for the next group to hit in front of you, and this is not continuous even though you are "walking." Keep in mind that the more you eat, the more intense your exercise and/or activities must be to just break even for losing weight. And remember, your activity days don't count the same as your exercise days when it comes to burning up calories, so if you eat the same amount on these days, you will not lose weight despite your good intentions.

TIPS TO CREATE A BETTER BALANCE

Although you are always exercising and moving, you can see that it is very difficult to be consistent with losing weight while applying this approach. Too many factors play into your success while allowing little room for error, especially if your lifestyle changes or your work/home schedule and responsibilities increase to the point that you find that you are not able to fit either exercise or your favorite activity in that day. When this occurs, you have to work out twice as long and twice as intensely in order to just break even with weight loss to compensate for those extra calories you consumed because you did not adjust and lower your caloric intake. Try some of the tips listed here to help lower your caloric intake and cut down on the number of days you are moving:

- Jot down on a piece of paper a typical week for you, separating the number of days you are active from the number of days you work out.

- Strive for five days of pure exercise and two days of activities.

- On your two active days, learn to discipline yourself and consume fewer calories.

- Take a cooking class and learn how to prepare your favorite dishes with low-fat and lower-calorie options.

- Drink lots of water 15–30 minutes before you eat dinner; you will feel full and this will help naturally to lower your urge to overeat and/or drink to excess.

- When you are hungry between meals, eat a piece of fruit instead of your normally high-fat and high-calorie foods.

- If you eat dessert often, cut down to two times a week or eat half-portions. In one week that will help you lose an extra pound or more.

- If you normally eat out for the majority of your meals, prepare your breakfast and lunch the night before and take them in to work with you. People who eat home-cooked prepared meals consume less fat and fewer calories because they can better *control* the fat and total calorie content of these foods.

- Choose more nonactive and passive-type hobbies and "rest" your body at least one day a week. If you have ever wanted to write a book or poetry, now is the time to start!

- Every three or four months, take a full week off from exercise and only practice mild-type activities. You will feel mentally and physically rested and will come back to your exercise regimen with a "renewed" vim and vigor. By resting your body like this, you will also lower your risk of injury.

- If you have a family and you are feeling "antsy" and must move, play and teach your child or children sports for a few hours. That way you are moving but in a passive rather than intense manner, so you at least have satisfied your need to be moving that day.

- Enroll in a yoga class one day per week and learn how to become more relaxed while increasing circulation, range of motion, and overall body flexibility.

In summary, your goal is to make small adjustments and go from seven days per week of exercise/activity to five days per week. At the same time, you want to decrease your total caloric intake by 25 to 35 percent over time. With time, as you begin to ingest less calories, you will soon realize that you can lose weight without having to move each and every day like a wild man or woman. And remember, as you age, your BMR slows down a little bit more each year, so if you are still eating the same amount now at 45 years old as you ate when you were 21 years old, even if you work out seven days a week you will still gain weight. And more important, you have left no room for error such as exercising or moving fewer days per week due to any change in your lifestyle.

Option #2, Balanced Approach—Weight Loss Through Maintaining Equilibrium

BACKGROUND AND PERSPECTIVE ON DIET AND EXERCISE

This is the "ideal" approach to losing weight and keeping it off for life. However, it is important to note that although many aspire to or actually follow this formula, they still fall way short of achieving their weight-loss goals primarily due to the fact that their exercise regimen is often flawed or on the days that they don't move they have a bad-eating day, thus creating a "double negative," which means that they need to have a "double positive day" just to get back to break-even status with their weight-loss regimen. You are fortunate that probably since childhood you learned to walk away from the dinner table or only ate until you felt full, rarely overeating. You also did not eat often or a lot between meals, knowing that you would eventually gain weight. You were active as a child and may have played organized sports, not necessarily because you loved them but more out of your parents' urging or perhaps for social reasons. You "diet" and exercise when you see that you've put on a few pounds, but never for too long, just long enough to shed that weight, and then both your diet and exercise go on a "hiatus." You could be classified at times as a yo-yo exerciser and yo-yo dieter, possessing enough smarts to lose weight when you feel like doing so. You are motivated to do so by perhaps a social event coming up when you fit snugly into a suit or dress, a romance, your image at work, or trying to look like your girlfriend or pal. Your problem has more to do with consistency and maintaining that regularity rather than the process itself. You know what to do, you just can't or, better yet, you choose not to do it all the time. Your weight fluctuates from being 10 to 20 pounds overweight depending upon the time of year and what you have going on with your life at that particular time.

You typically will lose weight to get the woman or man but, once you have her or him, you start ignoring your weight and don't feel the same urgency to exercise and eat properly. Which reminds me; why do we take better care of ourselves and tend to take more pride in the we way present ourselves to our potential mates up to the point of being in a relationship and once we get married or feel comfortable we no longer find it a priority to maintain our well-being? Getting the woman or landing your man is easy; it's keeping him/her that is important. I cannot tell you how many times a man or woman has come into Exude overweight, out-of-shape, telling me that now that he or she is divorced or is in the middle of a breakup it's time to get back in shape. So, what you're telling me, Ms. Smith or Mr. Jones, is that you only see or feel an obligation to yourself to get and keep in shape now that you are back in the hunt? I can assure you, there would be a lot fewer divorced couples out there if they did whatever it took to make themselves more presentable and attractive to their partners once they're in a relationship.

You also have a tendency to be "streaky" with exercise and eating properly, sometimes doing it for three to six months and then, out of nowhere, stopping for months on end as well. At times, you view it as something you have to do rather than something you want to do. One of the reasons that you don't exercise with consistency is because you use your work or "I'm too busy" as your rationale for not exercising. You loathe starving yourself or overexercising, and in between gigs you choose passive-type activities and exercises such as yoga, walking, ice-skating, tennis, skiing, or the like. This lack of intensity during your activity or exercise helps you very little in the way of burning sufficient calories to prevent you from gaining weight even though you are moving and exercising.

You have the potential to practice great discipline and demonstrate consistency with exercise and food but always fall way short of permanent weight loss because either it isn't important enough for you or you find it too tedious for your liking. That, coupled with the fact that you can always get "back on track," is your downfall as well as your "ace in the hole."

YOUR FITNESS AND DIET GAME PLAN

Unlike your counterparts, you don't necessarily need to create a better balance as much as you need to work on mimicking this behavior and balance of eating sensibly and exercising consistently with more intensity. Your need to focus on exercising with more intensity, thus burning off those calories, combined with learning to eat lighter on the days you are not moving or exercising.

TIPS TO CREATE A BETTER BALANCE

- Don't look at exercise and dieting as a chore; try to have a healthier attitude toward them both.

- Remember that you don't need to work out and diet in such a severe way if you just cut down on your eating a bit and exercise with more regularity and intensity.

- Instead of overindulging with food and lack of exercise on your inactive days, save your eating frenzies for the days you exercise, and with the proper intensity of course.

- Think of how great you feel when you do exercise and eat sensibly. Try to go to bed with that feeling in mind and make a promise to yourself to copy that behavior day after day.

- On days that you are experiencing more stress, either personal or work-related, really discipline yourself and make sure you exercise to help alleviate the stress. By doing so, you will tend to eat healthier and sleep better as well.

- Look at exercise as your "therapy and remedy" for combating your eating and drinking urges, depression, and mood swings.

- After a long day at work or at home, before you settle down for a drink, force yourself to go and exercise. That drink will taste like a million dollars.

- To ensure that you get your workouts in during your really hectic days, jot down on Fridays your exercise days for the upcoming week and overbook by one or two days so that when you cannot make one because of your work obligations, you'll have a couple tucked away for insurance purposes.

- Keep a food log during the times you are not exercising and compare your eating habits with those when you're working out. You'll easily see that on the days you exercise, your eating patterns are noticeably better.

In summary, in order for you to lose and keep losing weight, you want to strive for five days of exercise per week combined with eating sensibly six days per week. That one "bad" day of overindulging would you serve you better on an exercise day rather than a day when you are inactive.

Part II

On the one hand, no one can stick to any extreme diet for long periods of time without eventually deviating to satisfy his/her urges. On the other hand, there are also those of you who loathe exercise and cannot and will not work out five, six or seven days a week no matter what I tell you or what incentives I throw at you. During our childhood and adolescence and while being a young adult and as a full-grown adult we all formed certain patterns, likes, and dislikes regarding our eating and exercise habits. When it comes to weight loss, one thing is certain: we need to create a caloric deficit in order to lose weight. To be more successful at it long-term, the amount of calories we expend at the end of any given day *must be* greater than the amount of calories we've consumed for that particular day. It is a medical and scientific fact.

As I've already explained in the previous chapter, there are many ways and techniques that we can employ in order for this deficit to occur. This Escape Your Weight—Diet/Exercise Guide is designed for you to choose the weight-loss path that puts the least amount of stress on your mind and body. In other words, if you are used to dieting or prefer to diet more than exercise in order to achieve weight loss, then choose that plan and stick to it. Or, perhaps you'd rather exercise a bit more rather than diet to lose weight; choose that particular plan and you'll be successful as well. What's important is that whichever approach you choose, you follow the procedures for dieting and/or exercise *precisely* as outlined, thus ensuring that you'll attain permanent weight loss. I cannot overemphasize this. Too often, people pick and choose certain *elements* from a diet and/or exercise plan that they are willing to do rather than following it precisely to a T. It is for this reason that you will not achieve your weight-loss goals and this reason alone. You cannot arbitrarily decide what to do and/or what not to do if you want to become thinner. Besides, that's what you have been doing your entire life thus far, with little results.

I have written this book and these diet/exercise plans for you so that it takes the guesswork out of it. In twenty years of designing weight-loss programs, I have never witnessed or experienced an individual who had not successfully reached his/her weight-loss goals when he/she has done what I have asked him/her to do. The only time "it doesn't work" is when they're not *working*. By "working" I simply mean sticking to the plan! Whichever approach you choose, whether it be Limited, Dynamic, or Balanced, all you need to do is follow the diet and exercise prescriptions and you will win at weight loss.

You may switch your approach, but do not take elements from one approach and mix and match them like an a la carte menu: they are not designed to work that way and you will fail. So, when you begin your journey towards weight loss and start applying the principles within each approach, if you find yourself not losing as much weight as you should be, all you need to do is review in your mind what elements in your diet and/or exercise prescription you are not adhering to and you have your answer. Go back and give a better effort by being honest with yourself and regrouping and starting afresh.

Each weight-loss category is broken down with a precise diet and exercise regimen for you to follow. Based on the approach that you choose, make sure that you are only taking in the allotted amount of calories for the day matched up with the exercise regimen and frequency needed for you to lose and keep losing weight until you get to your desired weight. Once you've chosen your pill (approach) you can follow the next weight-loss category's diet and exercise routine that you feel most comfortable with to propel you toward your weight-loss goals.

There will be days when you simply cannot or will not adhere to either your diet and/or your exercise plan. It is a fact of life. The *key* to successful weight loss is to slowly replace these bad days with good days. This takes time, focus, and determination. More important, it must be a priority. Now that you are armed and educated and know what to do as well as what not to do, you control your own destiny. If you want to win at weight loss, you need to make and create this to be a priority; otherwise, you will not win. I want you to think back and reflect on any endeavor, be it personal or professional, that you have attempted and have not succeeded at. I bet the number of times you have failed had more to do with your effort or perhaps the approach you unwisely chose than with ability. In reality, it really boils down to effort, which is synonymous with priority. For whatever reason, it just wasn't important enough. As long as you are aware of this, you can alter your behavior and take a step back and think about what you need to do in order to make it important enough. And it doesn't matter what or why you choose to motivate yourself to start losing weight. Whether it is for health reasons, vanity, the ability to be more active, the desire for a new mate or simply because you cannot stand looking in the mirror, as long as you are willing to give the required effort you will win at weight loss. You do not need to substantiate anything to anyone, including yourself.

Good luck!

ESCAPE YOUR WEIGHT QUIZ

If you are not sure or are hesitant as to which of the three approaches to choose from in your quest for weight loss, please take the short quiz below:

When trying to lose weight, please circle one of the following you'd be more apt to do:

1. **Carefully watch your daily diet, sprinkled with a little exercise 1–2 days per week.**
2. **Make moderate changes to your diet combined with exercise 3–5 days per week.**
3. **Exercise often, 5–7 days per week, sprinkled with little changes to your diet.**

If you chose number 1, then you will be following the Limited Approach.

If you chose number 2, then you will be following the Balanced Approach.

If you chose number 3, then you will be following the Dynamic Approach.

Now that you have chosen the approach that is best suited to your everyday environment and lifestyle, please refer to the Diet/Exercise guide to find the right weight-loss formula outlined for you.

Escape Your Weight—The Diet/Exercise Guide

	Diet Frequency: # of Days/Week (Diet Needs to be Good)	Exercise Frequency: # of Days Need to Exercise	Intensity of Exercise: Low-Moderate-High	Type: Aerobic vs. Anaerobic Percent Time Spent During 60 Minutes of Exercise
Weight Loss 60 + lbs. **Limited (Red) Approach**	7	2	Low-Moderate	80–90 Percent Aerobic 10–20 Percent Anaerobic
Weight Loss 60 + lbs. **Balanced (Yellow) Approach**	5	4–5	Moderate	80–90 Percent Aerobic 10–20 Percent Anaerobic
Weight Loss 60 + lbs. **Dynamic (Green) Approach**	2	6–7	Moderate	80–90 Percent Aerobic 10–20 Percent Anaerobic
Weight Loss 31–60 lbs. **Limited (Red) Approach**	7	2	Moderate	70 Percent Aerobic 30 Percent Anaerobic
Weight Loss 31–60 lbs. **Balanced (Yellow) Approach**	5	4–5	Moderate-High	70 Percent Aerobic 30 Percent Anaerobic
Weight Loss 31–60 lbs. **Dynamic (Green) Approach**	3	6–7	Moderate	70 Percent Aerobic 30 Percent Anaerobic
Weight Loss 11–30 lbs. **Limited (Red) Approach**	7	2	Moderate	60 Percent Aerobic 40 Percent Anaerobic
Weight Loss 11–30 lbs. **Balanced (Yellow) Approach**	5	4–5	High	60 Percent Aerobic 40 Percent Anaerobic
Weight Loss 11–30 lbs. **Dynamic (Green) Approach**	4	6–7	Moderate	60 Percent Aerobic 40 Percent Anaerobic
Weight Loss 10 lbs. or less **Limited (Red) Approach**	7	2	High	50 Percent Aerobic 50 Percent Anaerobic
Weight Loss 10 lbs. or less **Balanced (Yellow) Approach**	6	4–5	High	50 Percent Aerobic 50 Percent Anaerobic
Weight Loss 10 lbs. or less **Dynamic (Green) Approach**	5	6–7	High	50 Percent Aerobic 50 Percent Anaerobic

CHAPTER FIVE

Plans for Losing 60 Pounds or More

Most Important Factor in Diet Plans

It is often more difficult for people who have been overweight a good part or their entire lives to see the light at the end of the tunnel. You have never seen the "in-shape" person that is hidden inside, and, as a result do not always recognize your potential when you view yourself in the mirror. Typically, you are also starting off with so many bad habits (often no exercise and poor eating) or have only attempted weight loss through severe "dieting," so it can be a bit overwhelming.

To be successful, it is vital to think about baby steps. Making just one small change at a time adds up to big differences in the long run. Start off each week with a plan to change something small about your eating patterns and habits . . . It could be as simple as adding in an extra salad or bringing in a healthier snack to work instead of perhaps skipping a meal, overeating, or making a poor selection when eating. While attempting to lose weight, by focusing on making small improvements one day at a time you will begin to develop better eating routines that eventually will become an instilled habit. Before you know it, that change will result in the scale's starting to go downwards, and with the synergy of regular exercise you are guaranteed to continue to lose weight and, little by little, you become a healthier person with a new and positive outlook about yourself.

Helpful Tips for Successful Weight Reduction:

Keep a Food Journal—Write down what and when you eat and drink in a day and why: The journal will help you become aware of what you eat, will increase your control over eating, and will help you become aware of your eating patterns. Food becomes fattening when it is eaten for entertainment, comfort, or stress reduction.

Become Aware of Meal Timing: Eating earlier in the day prevents you from getting too hungry, losing control, and overeating in the evening.

Learn Your Calorie Budget: Know how much you can eat and still lose weight so you can be sure to fuel your body with an adequate amount of essential nutrients.

Eat Slowly: The brain needs about 20 minutes to receive the signal that you've eaten your fill. Practice by putting your fork down between bites and taking pauses throughout the meal.

Keep Away from Food Sources That Tempt You: Out of sight, out of mind, out of *mouth!* Hide high-calorie foods and keep healthy snacks readily available.

*Please note: For those individuals who are vegetarian or have other special dietary needs, please log on to eatright.org or ediets.com to find a dietician near you.

Meal Plans for Losing 60 Pounds or More

Limited Approach
1800 CALORIES PER DAY
(247 GM CARBOHYDRATE, 90 GM PROTEIN, 50 GM FAT)

BREAKFAST *(600 calories, approx. 82 gm carbohydrate, 30 gm protein, 16 gm fat):*

1. (600 calories, 82 gm carb, 28 gm protein, 15 gm fat)

    2 1/4 cups whole grain cereal (unsweetened, ready-to-eat cereal)

    1 1/2 cups skim milk

    1 1/4 cups berries

    12 almonds

    1 hard-boiled egg

2. (600 calories, 85 gm carb, 36 gm protein, 17 gm fat)

    1/2 cup 1 percent cottage cheese

    1 cup berries

    1 cup melon

    1/3 cup Grape-Nuts

    12 almonds

    1 slice of whole grain bread

    2 tsps. peanut butter

3. (600 calories, 82 gm carb, 29 gm protein, 15 gm fat)

   2 slices of whole grain bread

   1 tbsp. peanut butter

   1 apple

   12 oz. low-fat yogurt

   1/2 cup low-fat granola

4. (600 calories, 80 gm carb, 28 gm protein, 15 gm fat)

   2 poached eggs

   2 slices of whole grain bread

   3/4 cup plain low-fat yogurt

   1 1/2 cups melon

   1 cup mixed berries

5. (600 calories, 78 gm carb, 33 gm protein, 15 gm fat)

   2 cups cooked oatmeal

   12 chopped walnut halves

1 chopped Red Delicious apple

3/4 cup low-fat cottage cheese

6. (600 calories, 80 gm carb, 27 gm protein, 15 gm fat)

   Omelet—2 whole eggs + 1/2 oz. of low-fat cheese + 1/2 cup spinach + 1/2 cup chopped tomato

   2 slices of whole grain bread

   1 cup sliced strawberries

   1 sliced kiwi

   1 cup cubed melon

7. (600 calories, 84 gm carb, 30 gm protein, 16 gm fat)

   2 slices of whole grain bread

   2 oz. cheese

   1/2 cup sliced tomato

   2 1/2 cups mixed melon

   1 cup skim milk

LUNCH *(600 calories, approx. 82 gm carbohydrate, 30 gm protein, 16 gm fat):*

1. (600 calories, 80 gm carb, 29 gm protein, 15 gm fat)

   2 slices of whole grain bread

   3 oz. white meat turkey

   1/4 avocado

   1/2 cup sliced tomato and lettuce

   1 cup unsweetened apple
   sauce with 1/4 cup low-fat granola

2. (600 calories, 80 gm carb, 29 gm protein, 15 gm fat)

   1 whole wheat pita

   3 oz. chunk white tuna fish

3 tsps. mayonnaise

1/2 cup mixed shredded carrots, lettuce, and celery

36 cherries

3. (600 calories, 80 gm carb, 29 gm protein, 15 gm fat)

   3 oz. of cold chicken (cut up), mixed with 3 tsps. mayonnaise

   2 slices of rye bread

   1/2 cup sliced tomato and lettuce

   1 whole diced mango

   1 cup raspberries

4. (600 calories, 80 gm carb, 35 gm protein, 15 gm fat)

    Big Salad:

    2 cups mixed greens

    1/2 cup diced carrots

    1/2 cup diced bell peppers

    1/3 cup beans

    3 oz. grilled chicken

    4 chopped walnuts

    1 diced apple

    2 tbsps. vinaigrette salad dressing

    1 medium nectarine

    6-inch whole wheat pita

5. (600 calories, 85 gm carb, 31 gm protein, 15 gm fat)

    3 oz. lean roast beef

    2 slices rye bread

    1 tsp. mayonnaise

    1/2 cup sliced tomato and lettuce

    1/2 cup carrot sticks

    1 1/2 cups fresh pineapple + 1 cup diced

papaya topped with 6 slivered almonds

6. (600 calories, 80 gm carb, 30 gm protein, 15 gm fat)

    3 cups spinach

    1 oz. feta cheese

    1 oz. firm tofu

    1/2 cup water chestnuts

    1/2 cup snap peas

    1 1/2 cups mandarin oranges

    1 tbsp. reduced-fat ginger salad dressing

    10 whole grain crackers

7. (600 calories, 80 gm carb, 31 gm protein, 15 gm fat)

    2 slices of whole grain bread

    2 oz. white meat turkey

    1 oz. low-fat cheese

    2 tsps. mayonnaise

    1/2 cup sliced tomato and lettuce

    1 1/2 cups mixed fruit salad

    3 whole-wheat graham crackers

DINNER *(600 calories, approx. 82 gm carbohydrate, 30 gm protein, 16 gm fat):*

1. (600 calories, 85 gm carb, 28 gm protein, 15 gm fat)

    2 oz. cooked chicken (no skin)

    1 cup brown rice

    1 cup green beans sautéed in 1 tsp. olive oil and 6 slivered almonds

    1 cup mixed greens with 1/2 cup chopped tomatoes and 1/2 cup chopped peppers

    1 tbsp. salad dressing

    1 medium apple

2. (600 calories, 85 gm carb, 26 gm protein, 16 gm fat)

    2 oz. lean cooked roast beef

    2/3 cup brown rice

    1/2 cup carrots

    1/2 cup cauliflower

    2 tsps. olive oil

1 whole grain dinner roll

1 orange

3. (600 calories, 83 gm carb, 29 gm protein, 16 gm fat)

   2 oz. broiled salmon

   1 large sweet potato

   1 cup sautéed spinach with 2 tsps. olive oil

   1 cup sliced tomato

   1 1/2 cups diced melon

4. (600 calories, 85 gm carb, 30 gm protein, 16 gm fat)

   2 oz. sautéed shrimp in 2 tsps. olive oil

   1 1/2 cups whole wheat pasta

   1 1/2 cup jarred tomato sauce

   1 1/2 cup artichoke hearts

   1 1/2 cup spinach

   1 1/4 cups sliced strawberries

   1 sliced fresh peach

5. (600 calories, 80 gm carb, 32 gm protein, 16 gm fat)

3 oz. baked cod

1/3 cup cooked whole wheat couscous

2 cups baked winter squash

1 cup mixed greens (kale, collard, and mustard) sautéed in 3 tsps. olive oil

2 cups cubed papaya

6. (600 calories, 85 gm carb, 27 gm protein, 16 gm fat)

   2 oz. flank steak

   1 cup whole wheat couscous

   2 cups roasted broccoli and cauliflower with 2 tsps. olive oil

   1 1/2 cups raspberries

7. (500 calories, 83 gm carb, 27 gm protein, 16 gm fat)

   2 oz. barbecued chicken

   1 medium corn on the cob

   1 cup baked beans

   1 1/2 cups cucumber and tomato salad tossed with 2 tbsps. olive oil–based dressing

   1/2 cup cubed watermelon

Dynamic Approach
2200 CALORIES PER DAY
(274 GM CARBOHYDRATE, 110 GM PROTEIN, 60 GM FAT)

BREAKFAST *(600 calories, approx. 82 gm carbohydrate, 30 gm protein, 16 gm fat):*

1. (600 calories, 82 gm carb, 28 gm protein, 15 gm fat)

   2 1/4 cups whole grain cereal (unsweetened, ready-to-eat cereal)

   1 1/2 cup skim milk

   1 1/4 cups berries

12 almonds

1 hard-boiled egg

2. (600 calories, 85 gm carb, 36 gm protein, 17 gm fat)

   1/2 cup 1 percent cottage cheese

1 cup berries

1 cup melon

$^{1}/_{3}$ cup Grape-Nuts

12 almonds

1 slice of whole grain bread

2 tsps. peanut butter

3. (600 calories, 82 gm carb, 29 gm protein,
   15 gm fat)

   2 slices of whole grain bread

   1 tsp. peanut butter

   1 apple

   12 oz. low-fat yogurt

   $^{1}/_{2}$ cup low-fat granola

4. (600 calories, 80 gm carb, 28 gm protein,
   15 gm fat)

   2 poached eggs

   2 slices of whole grain bread

   $^{3}/_{4}$ cup plain low-fat yogurt

   1 $^{1}/_{2}$ cups melon

   1 cup mixed berries

5. (600 calories, 78 gm carb, 33 gm protein,
   15 gm fat)

   2 cups cooked oatmeal

   12 chopped walnut halves

   1 chopped Red Delicious apple

   $^{3}/_{4}$ cup low-fat cottage cheese

6. (600 calories, 80 gm carb, 27 gm protein,
   15 gm fat)

   Omelet—2 whole eggs + $^{1}/_{2}$ oz. of low-fat
       cheese + $^{1}/_{2}$ cup spinach + $^{1}/_{2}$ cup
       chopped tomato

   2 slices of whole grain bread

   1 cup sliced strawberries

   1 sliced kiwi

   1 cup cubed melon

7. (600 calories, 84 gm carb, 30 gm protein,
   16 gm fat)

   2 slices of whole grain bread

   2 oz. cheese

   $^{1}/_{2}$ cup sliced tomato

   2 $^{1}/_{2}$ cups mixed melon

   1 cup skim milk

SNACK *(200 calories, approx. 27 gm carbohydrate, 10 gm protein, 6 gm fat):*

1. (200 calories, 27 gm carb, 8 gm protein,
   5 gm fat)

   1 cup plain nonfat yogurt

   $^{3}/_{4}$ cup fresh blackberries

   6 chopped almonds

2. (200 calories, 27 gm carb, 8 gm protein,
   5 gm fat)

1 medium apple

2 tsps. peanut butter

1 cup skim milk

3. (200 calories, 30 gm carb, 7 gm protein,
   7 gm fat)

   1 whole grain English muffin

   1 oz. Swiss cheese

4. (200 calories, 27 gm carb, 8 gm protein, 5 gm fat)

   Peanut-butter-and-jelly smoothie: Blend 1 cup skim milk + 1¼ cups fresh or frozen strawberries + 2 tsps. peanut butter

5. (200 calories, 27 gm carb, 8 gm protein, 5 gm fat)

   six-inch whole wheat pita

   1 sliced apple

   2 tsps. peanut butter

6. (200 calories, 27 gm carb, 8 gm protein, 5 gm fat)

   1 slice whole wheat raisin bread topped with 1 sliced kiwi and ¼ cup ricotta cheese

7. (200 calories, 27 gm carb, 8 gm protein, 5 gm fat)

   ½ six-inch whole wheat pita

   ⅓ cup hummus

   ½ cup carrot sticks

LUNCH *(600 calories, approx. 82 gm carbohydrate, 30 gm protein, 16 gm fat):*

1. (600 calories, 80 gm carb, 29 gm protein, 15 gm fat)
   2 slices of whole grain bread
   3 oz. white meat turkey
   ¼ avocado
   ½ cup sliced tomato and lettuce
   1 cup unsweetened applesauce with ¼ cup low-fat granola

2. (600 calories, 80 gm carb, 29 gm protein, 15 gm fat)
   1 whole wheat pita
   3 oz. chunk white tuna fish
   3 tsps. mayonnaise
   ½ cup mixed shredded carrots, lettuce, and celery
   36 cherries

3. (600 calories, 80 gm carb, 29 gm protein, 15 gm fat)
   3 oz. of cold chicken (cut up) mixed with 3 tsps. mayonnaise
   2 slices of rye bread

   ½ cup sliced tomato and lettuce
   1 whole diced mango
   1 cup raspberries

4. (600 calories, 80 gm carb, 35 gm protein, 15 gm fat)
   Big Salad:
   2 cups mixed greens
   ½ cup diced carrots
   ½ cup diced bell peppers
   ⅓ cup beans
   3 oz. grilled chicken
   4 chopped walnuts
   1 diced apple
   2 tbsps. vinaigrette salad dressing
   1 medium nectarine
   6-inch whole wheat pita

5. (600 calories, 85 gm carb, 31 gm protein, 15 gm fat)
   3 oz. lean roast beef

2 slices of rye bread

1 tsp. mayonnaise

1/2 cup sliced tomato and lettuce

1/2 cup carrot sticks

1 1/2 cup fresh pineapple + 1 cup diced
    papaya topped with 6 slivered almonds

6. (600 calories, 80 gm carb, 30 gm protein,
   15 gm fat)

3 cups spinach

1 oz. feta cheese

1 oz. firm tofu

1/2 cup water chestnuts

1/2 cup snap peas

1 1/2 cups mandarin oranges

1 tbsp. reduced-fat ginger salad dressing

10 whole grain crackers

7. (600 calories, 80 gm carb, 31 gm protein,
   15 gm fat)

2 slices of whole grain bread

2 oz. white meat turkey

1 oz. low-fat cheese

2 tsps. mayonnaise

1/2 cup sliced tomato and lettuce

1 1/2 cups mixed fruit salad

3 whole wheat graham crackers

SNACK *(200 calories, approx. 27 gm carbohydrate, 10 gm protein, 6 gm fat):*

1. (200 calories, 27 gm carb, 8 gm protein,
   5 gm fat)

   1 cup plain nonfat yogurt

   3/4 cup fresh blackberries

   6 chopped almonds

2. (200 calories, 27 gm carb, 8 gm protein,
   5 gm fat)

   1 medium apple

   2 tsps. peanut butter

   1 cup skim milk

3. (200 calories, 30 gm carb, 7 gm protein,
   7 gm fat)

   1 whole grain English muffin

   1 oz. Swiss cheese

4. (200 calories, 27 gm carb, 8 gm protein,
   5 gm fat)

   Peanut-butter-and-jelly smoothie: Blend 1
       cup skim milk + 1 1/4 cups fresh or
       frozen strawberries + 2 tsps. peanut
       butter

5. (200 calories, 27 gm carb, 8 gm protein,
   5 gm fat)

   six-inch whole wheat pita

   1 sliced apple

   2 tsps. peanut butter

6. (200 calories, 27 gm carb, 8 gm protein,
   5 gm fat)

   1 slice whole wheat raisin bread topped with
       1 sliced kiwi and 1/4 cup ricotta cheese

7. (200 calories, 27 gm carb, 8 gm protein, 5 gm fat)

   1/2 six-inch whole wheat pita

   1/3 cup hummus

   1/2 cup carrot sticks

DINNER *(600 calories, approx. 82 gm carbohydrate, 30 gm protein, 16 gm fat):*

1. (600 calories, 85 gm carb, 28 gm protein, 15 gm fat)

   2 oz. cooked chicken (no skin)

   1 cup brown rice

   1 cup green beans sautéed in 1 tsp. olive oil and 6 slivered almonds

   1 cup mixed greens with 1/2 cup chopped tomatoes and 1/2 cup chopped peppers

   1 tbsp. salad dressing

   1 medium apple

2. (600 calories, 85 gm carb, 26 gm protein, 16 gm fat)

   2 oz. lean cooked roast beef

   2/3 cup brown rice

   1/2 cup carrots

   1/2 cup cauliflower

   2 tsps. olive oil

   1 whole grain dinner roll

   1 orange

3. (600 calories, 83 gm carb, 29 gm protein, 16 gm fat)

   2 oz. broiled salmon

   1 large sweet potato

   1 cup sautéed spinach with 2 tsps. olive oil

   1 cup sliced tomato

   1 1/2 cups diced melon

4. (600 calories, 85 gm carb, 30 gm protein, 16 gm fat)

   2 oz. sautéed shrimp in 2 tsps. olive oil

   1 1/2 cups whole wheat pasta

   1/2 cup jarred tomato sauce

   1/2 cup artichoke hearts

   1/2 cup spinach

   1 1/4 cups sliced strawberries

   1 sliced fresh peach

5. (600 calories, 80 gm carb, 32 gm protein, 16 gm fat)

   3 oz. baked cod

   1/3 cup cooked whole wheat couscous

   2 cups baked winter squash

   1 cup mixed greens (kale, collard, and mustard) sautéed in 3 tsps. olive oil

   2 cups cubed papaya

6. (600 calories, 85 gm carb, 27 gm protein, 16 gm fat)

   2 oz. flank steak

   1 cup whole wheat couscous

   2 cups roasted broccoli and cauliflower with 2 tsps. olive oil

   1 1/2 cups raspberries

7. (500 calories, 83 gm carb, 27 gm protein, 16 gm fat)

   2 oz. barbecued chicken

   1 medium corn on the cob

1 cup baked beans

1 1/2 cups cucumber and tomato salad

tossed with 2 tbsps. olive oil–based dressing

1/2 cup cubed watermelon

Balanced Approach

2000 CALORIES PER DAY

(274 GM CARBOHYDRATE, 98 GM PROTEIN, 56 GM FAT)

BREAKFAST *(600 calories, approx. 82 gm carbohydrate, 30 gm protein, 16 gm fat)*:

1. (600 calories, 82 gm carb, 28 gm protein, 15 gm fat)

   2 1/4 cups whole grain cereal (unsweetened, ready-to-eat cereal),

   1 1/2 cups skim milk

   1 1/4 cups berries

   12 almonds

   1 hard-boiled egg

2. (600 calories, 85 gm carb, 36 gm protein, 17 gm fat)

   1/2 cup 1 percent cottage cheese

   1 cup berries

   1 cup melon

   1/3 cup Grape-Nuts

   12 almonds

   1 slice of whole grain bread

   2 tsps. peanut butter

3. (600 calories, 82 gm carb, 29 gm protein, 15 gm fat)

   2 slices of whole grain bread

   1 tbsp. peanut butter

   1 apple

   12 oz. low-fat yogurt

   1/2 cup low-fat granola

4. (600 calories, 80 gm carb, 28 gm protein, 15 gm fat)

   2 poached eggs

   2 slices of whole grain bread

   3/4 cup plain low-fat yogurt

   1 1/2 cups melon

   1 cup mixed berries

5. (600 calories, 78 gm carb, 33 gm protein, 15 gm fat)

   2 cups cooked oatmeal

   12 chopped walnut halves

   1 chopped Red Delicious apple

   3/4 cup low-fat cottage cheese

6. (600 calories, 80 gm carb, 27 gm protein, 15 gm fat)

   Omelet—2 whole eggs + 1/2 oz. of low-fat cheese + 1/2 cup spinach + 1/2 cup chopped tomato

   2 slices of whole grain bread

   1 cup sliced strawberries

   1 sliced kiwi

   1 cup cubed melon

7. (600 calories, 84 gm carb, 30 gm protein, 16 gm fat)

2 slices of whole grain bread

2 oz. cheese

1/2 cup sliced tomato

2 1/2 cups mixed melon

1 cup skim milk

LUNCH *(600 calories, approx. 82 gm carbohydrate, 30 gm protein, 16 gm fat):*

1. (600 calories, 80 gm carb, 29 gm protein,
   15 gm fat)

   2 slices of whole grain bread

   3 oz. white meat turkey

   1/4 avocado

   1/2 cup sliced tomato and lettuce

   1 cup unsweetened applesauce with
      1/4 cup low-fat granola

2. (600 calories, 80 gm carb, 29 gm protein,
   15 gm fat)

   1 whole wheat pita

   3 oz. chunk white tuna fish

   3 tsps. mayonnaise

   1/2 cup mixed shredded carrots, lettuce, and
      celery

   36 cherries

3. (600 calories, 80 gm carb, 29 gm protein,
   15 gm fat)

   3 oz. of cold chicken (cut up) mixed with 3
      tsps. mayonnaise

   2 slices of rye bread

   1/2 cup sliced tomato and lettuce

   1 whole diced mango

   1 cup raspberries

4. (600 calories, 80 gm carb, 35 gm protein,
   15 gm fat)

   Big Salad:

2 cups mixed greens

1/2 cup diced carrots

1/2 cup diced bell peppers

1/3 cup beans

3 oz. grilled chicken

4 chopped walnuts

1 diced apple

2 tbsps. vinaigrette salad dressing

1 medium nectarine

six-inch whole wheat pita

5. (600 calories, 85 gm carb, 31 gm protein,
   15 gm fat)

   3 oz. lean roast beef

   2 slices of rye bread

   1 tsp. mayonnaise

   1/2 cup sliced tomato and lettuce

   1/2 cup carrot sticks

   1 1/2 cups fresh pineapple + 1 cup diced
      papaya topped with 6 slivered almonds

6. (600 calories, 80 gm carb, 30 gm protein,
   15 gm fat)

   3 cups spinach

   1 oz. feta cheese

   1 oz. firm tofu

   1/2 cup water chestnuts

   1/2 cup snap peas

   1 1/2 cups mandarin oranges

1 tbsp. reduced-fat ginger salad dressing

10 whole grain crackers

7. (600 calories, 80 gm carb, 31 gm protein, 15 gm fat)

2 slices of whole grain bread

2 oz. white meat turkey

1 oz. low-fat cheese

2 tsps. mayonnaise

1/2 cup sliced tomato and lettuce

1 1/2 cups mixed fruit salad

3 whole wheat graham crackers

SNACK *(200 calories, approx. 27 gm carbohydrate, 10 gm protein, 6 gm fat):*

1. (200 calories, 27 gm carb, 8 gm protein, 5 gm fat)

1 cup plain nonfat yogurt

3/4 cup fresh blackberries

6 chopped almonds

2. (200 calories, 27 gm carb, 8 gm protein, 5 gm fat)

1 medium apple

2 tsps. peanut butter

1 cup skim milk

3. (200 calories, 30 gm carb, 7 gm protein, 7 gm fat)

1 whole grain English muffin

1 oz. Swiss cheese

4. (200 calories, 27 gm carb, 8 gm protein, 5 gm fat)

Peanut-butter-and-jelly smoothie: Blend 1 cup skim milk + 1 1/4 cups fresh or frozen strawberries + 2 tsps. peanut butter

5. (200 calories, 27 gm carb, 8 gm protein, 5 gm fat)

six-inch whole wheat pita

1 sliced apple

2 tsps. peanut butter

6. (200 calories, 27 gm carb, 8 gm protein, 5 gm fat)

1 slice whole wheat raisin bread topped with 1 sliced kiwi and 1/4 cup ricotta cheese

7. (200 calories, 27 gm carb, 8 gm protein, 5 gm fat)

1/2 six-inch whole wheat pita

1/3 cup hummus

1/2 cup carrot sticks

DINNER *(600 calories, approx. 82 gm carbohydrate, 30 gm protein, 16 gm fat):*

1. (600 calories, 85 gm carb, 28 gm protein, 15 gm fat)

2 oz. cooked chicken (no skin)

1 cup brown rice

1 cup green beans sautéed in 1 tsp. olive oil and 6 slivered almonds

1 cup mixed greens with 1/2 cup chopped
    tomatoes and 1/2 cup chopped peppers

1 tbsp. salad dressing

1 medium apple

2. (600 calories, 85 gm carb, 26 gm protein, 16 gm fat)

    2 oz. lean cooked roast beef

    2/3 cup brown rice

    1/2 cup carrots

    1/2 cup cauliflower

    2 tsps. olive oil

    1 whole grain dinner roll

    1 orange

3. (600 calories, 83 gm carb, 29 gm protein, 16 gm fat)

    2 oz. broiled salmon

    1 large sweet potato

    1 cup sautéed spinach with 2 tsps. olive oil

    1 cup sliced tomato

    1 1/2 cups diced melon

4. (600 calories, 85 gm carb, 30 gm protein, 16 gm fat)

    2 oz. sautéed shrimp in 2 tsps. olive oil

    1 1/2 cups whole wheat pasta

    1/2 cup jarred tomato sauce

    1/2 cup artichoke hearts

1/2 cup spinach

1 1/4 cups sliced strawberries

1 sliced fresh peach

5. (600 calories, 80 gm carb, 32 gm protein, 16 gm fat)

    3 oz. baked cod

    1/3 cup cooked whole wheat couscous

    2 cups baked winter squash

    1 cup mixed greens (kale, collard, and mustard) sautéed in 3 tsps. olive oil

    2 cups cubed papaya

6. (600 calories, 85 gm carb, 27 gm protein, 16 gm fat)

    2 oz. flank steak

    1 cup whole wheat couscous

    2 cups roasted broccoli and cauliflower with 2 tsps. olive oil

    1 1/2 cups raspberries

7. (500 calories, 83 gm carb, 27 gm protein, 16 gm fat)

    2 oz. barbecued chicken

    1 medium corn on the cob

    1 cup baked beans

    1 1/2 cups cucumber and tomato salad tossed with 2 tbsps. olive oil–based dressing

    1/2 cup cubed watermelon

Additional Foods to Choose as Between Meal Snacks

LOW-CALORIE

Fresh fruit

Fresh vegetables (can dip them in 2 tbsps. hummus, salsa, or homemade low-fat dip)

Low-fat yogurt

Low-fat cottage cheese

Hot-air-popped popcorn

MEDIUM-CALORIE

1/4 cup dry-roasted nuts (need to limit portions)

1 tbsp. nut butter on a slice of whole wheat bread

1 tbsp. nut butter on a medium apple

2 tsps. peanut butter + 2 graham crackers + 2 tsps. jam

1 oz. of reduced-fat cheese with 10 whole grain crackers

1 slice of reduced-fat cheese melted over tomato on whole grain bread

Nonfat Greek yogurt with 1 cup of berries and 2 tbsps. chopped nuts

1/4 cup dry-roasted mixed nuts (almonds, pumpkinseeds, walnuts)

1/2 whole wheat English muffin + 1 slice low-fat mozzarella cheese + 1 tbsp. marinara sauce

1 medium orange diced into 1 serving of oatmeal + 2 walnut halves

FOR SWEET CRAVINGS

Fresh watermelon

Fresh berries

Sugar-free Jell-O

Fat-free/sugar-free fudge pop

Sugar-free Popsicle

FOR SAVORY CRAVINGS

Fresh vegetables dipped in salsa

Hot-air-popped popcorn

Exercise Prescription for Losing 60 Pounds or More

Most Important Factor

The most important element and differentiator as you propel yourself toward your weight-loss goals is your *frequency of workouts*. Your ultimate goal is to create an environment that allows you to exercise aerobically, 5× week. Depending upon which approach you decide to take with your weight-loss plan, simply put, the more you exercise the faster you will shed weight *without* having to severely restrict your food intake.

Fitness Equipment Needed

1. **Choose One:** Recumbent or upright stationary bike, treadmill, elliptical machine or cross trainer or, if no access to a piece of aerobic fitness equipment, walk instead
2. Firm exercise mat

3. A lightweight (2–4 lb.) collapsible aerobic toning bar for both men and women
4. Trampoline (optional)

(See page III for photos of fitness equipment needed.)

Please Note: All of the following exercise regimens can be performed at home, at the gym, or even while traveling.

Exercise Regimen

Frequency—2, 3, 4, or 5 days per week

Duration—40 to 60 minutes, depending upon your current level of fitness

**Before starting this or any exercise regimen, get your doctor's approval.

Workout #1

Full-Body Routine—2 to 3 days per week, every other day, Mondays, Wednesdays, and Fridays or Tuesdays, Thursdays, and Saturdays

"Reps" = Repetitions; the number of times you actually perform the exercise.

1. **Warm-up**—bike, brisk walk, elliptical or cross trainer for 20 minutes, using low resistance, 70 + RPMs or 3.0 + MPH while walking, with no incline.

   Please Note: If you are unable to perform 20 minutes of continuous aerobic exercise, take breaks for a minute or so, catch your breath, and resume until you have performed 20 minutes.

2. **Stretch**—4 minutes.

3. **Fat Burner**—5 minutes of biking or other aerobic piece, bouncing on trampoline, or walking.

4. **Stand-ups**—5 to 7 reps.

5. **Abdominals**—(a) knees to chest: 15 reps, rest 30 seconds, repeat 12 reps; (b) elbows to knees: 15 reps, rest 30 seconds, repeat 12 reps.

6. **Legs/Hips**—march in place: 30 to 50 reps.

7. **Fat Burner**—5 minutes of biking or other aerobic piece, bouncing on trampoline, or walking.

8. **Stand-ups**—5 to 7 reps.

9. **Upper Body Exercises**—with aerobic toning bar: (a) push-outs: 25 reps; (b) kick-backs: 25 reps.

10. **Fat Burner**—5 minutes of biking or other aerobic piece, bouncing on trampoline, or walking.

11. **Cooldown**—bike or walk for 3 minutes, nice and easy.

If you need a break at any time during your exercise regimen, you can simply get on a stationary bike or any other piece of aerobic equipment or walk 1–3 minutes to allow your heart rate to come down safely before you resume.

Based upon your current level of fitness, you can either increase or decrease the number of repetitions with each exercise. You should be progressing every two weeks by increasing the speed at which you bike or walk, et cetera, and increase your repetitions by 1–2 repetitions every 2 weeks for every exercise, trying to eventually get to 50 repetitions for each exercise. Also, if you can only perform a few repetitions of any exercise, don't skip it, do what you can do, because as you increase your frequency, the number of repetitions will increase as your fitness level improves.

Workout #2 (Optional, depending upon which approach you choose: Balanced or Dynamic)

Off Day Routine—2 to 3 days per week on days in between Full-Body Routines. To see instructions and view photos of stretches for your Off Day Routine, see pages 112–115.

1. Bike, brisk walk, elliptical machine or cross trainer for 30 minutes, moderate intensity.

2. Stretch—4 minutes.

3. Cooldown—3 minutes of easy biking or walking.

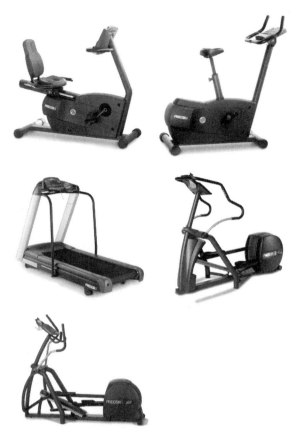

1. Aerobic Equipment

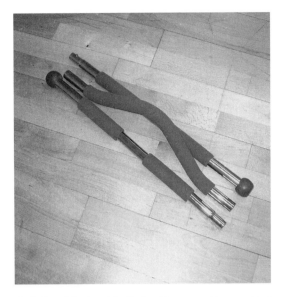

3. Collapsible Aerobic Toning Bar   Unassembled

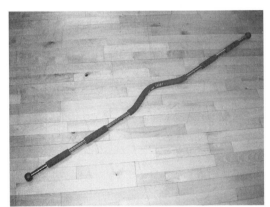

Assembled

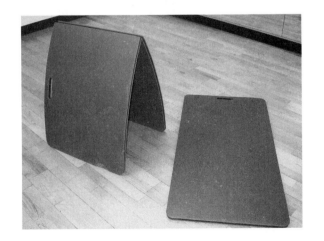

2. Firm Exercise Mat

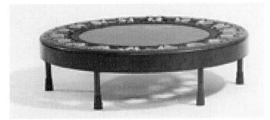

4. Trampoline

Workout #1–Full-Body Routine

1. Warm-up–20 minutes
2. Stretch—Hold each stretch for 30–60 seconds.

ARM CIRCLES

With arms outstretched, slowly circle your arms backward for 5 revolutions and then forward for 5 revolutions.

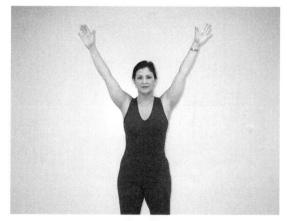

TRICEPS

With arms overhead, gently pull the left elbow behind your head with your right hand. Hold when you reach a comfortable stretch in the rear shoulder and upper back. Switch arms and repeat.

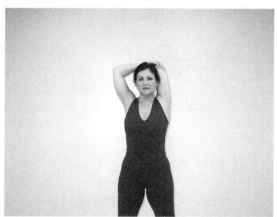

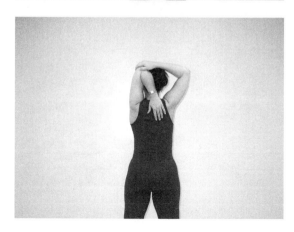

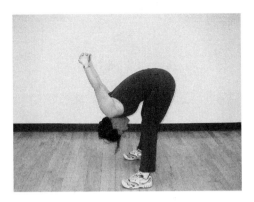

SHOULDERS, CHEST, AND HAMSTRINGS

Grasp hands behind your back, with palms facing each other. Slightly bend your knees and lift arms up as you bend forward at the waist. Hold when you feel a comfortable stretch in the shoulders, chest, and hamstrings.

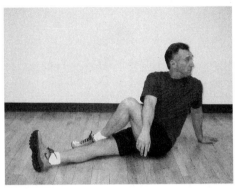

SPINAL TWIST

Keeping the right leg straight, left arm behind for support, cross left leg over and place foot outside the right knee. With the right hand or elbow on the left knee, slowly twist and look over your left shoulder while simultaneously pulling the knee in the opposite direction; hold. You will feel pressure in the hip, side, and upper back. Repeat on opposite side.

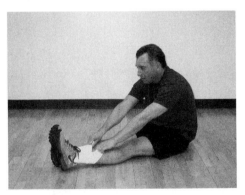

HAMSTRINGS

With legs straight, ankles flexed, bend forward from the hips and reach out toward your toes and, based on your flexibility, grab on to either your socks, shoelaces, or toes and hold the stretch. You will feel tension just behind the knees, in your upper calves, and in the lower back area.

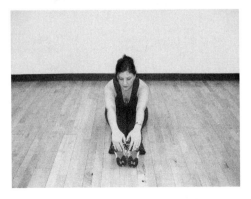

GROIN

In sitting position, pull the soles of your feet together and grab hold of your ankles. Gently pull heels toward the groin area. Let your knees relax toward the floor, and gently press your elbows down on your knees to increase the stretch.

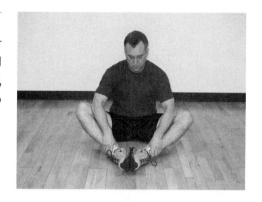

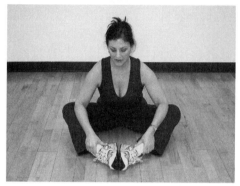

QUADRICEPS

Lie down on your left side. Bend your right leg back and grab your right ankle with your right hand. Gently pull your leg back toward your buttocks. Hold the position when you feel a comfortable stretch in front of your right thigh. Release slowly and roll over to your left side and repeat.

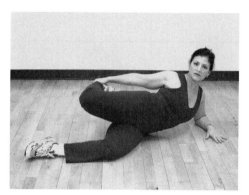

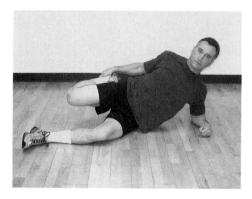

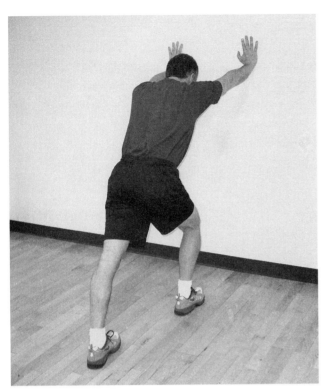

CALVES

Stand a little farther than arms' length away from a wall or solid support; lean on it with hands placed shoulder distance apart. Bring one foot forward, knee bent, while keeping the back leg straight, heel pressing into the floor. Lean toward wall while holding stretch. Switch legs and repeat.

3. **Fat Burner**—5 minutes of biking or other aerobic piece, bouncing on trampoline, or walking.

4. **Stand-ups**—may be performed with or without firm exercise mat.

STAND-UPS FROM THE FLOOR—5 to 7 reps

**Keep in mind that you may want to be next to a wall or stable surface such as a couch or chair for the stand-ups.

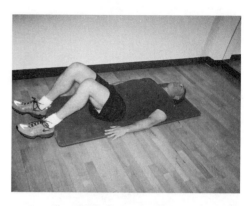

a. Lie on back with knees bent and heels on the floor.

b. Press yourself up into a seated position keeping knees bent.

c. Come onto hands and knees and place your right foot flat on the floor with your weight on your left knee, keeping back straight.

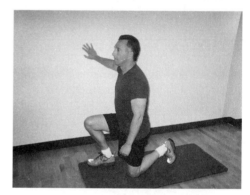

d. Get your balance; if needed, place your right hand on the wall or other stable surface as you push yourself up to a standing position.

e. Return to starting position and repeat by facing opposite direction and stand up by placing your left hand on the wall and keep alternating sides for each repetition throughout entire exercise.

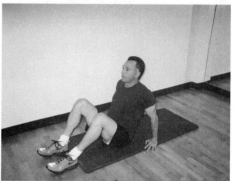

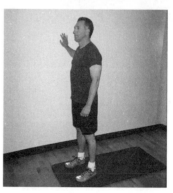

5. Abdominals–to be performed on a firm exercise mat.

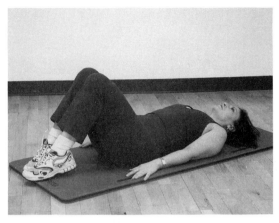

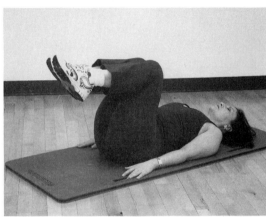

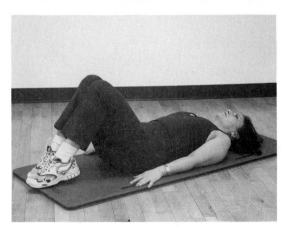

(a) KNEES TO CHEST–15 reps/12 reps

Lie on back with arms extended, hands next to buttocks, palms down. Raise knees and feet in a tucked position toward chest, keeping lower back pressed against the floor while exhaling. Lower feet to ground while inhaling and repeat. Keep upper half of body motionless throughout movement.

(b) ELBOWS TO KNEES—15 reps/12 reps

Lying on back, raise knees and feet toward chest in a tucked position. Clasp your hands at the base of your neck. Gently curl your upper body, bringing your elbows toward your knees while exhaling. Slowly lower back and shoulders to ground while inhaling and repeat. Keep lower body motionless throughout entire movement.

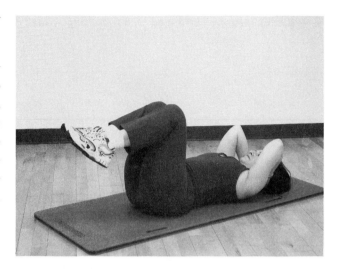

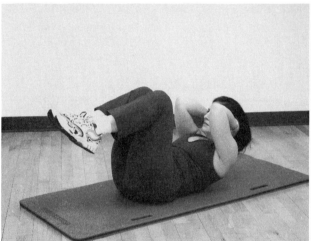

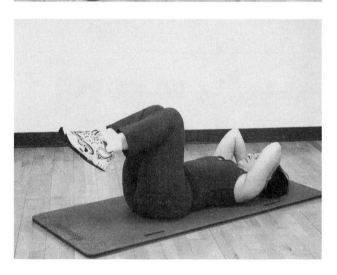

6. Legs/Hips.

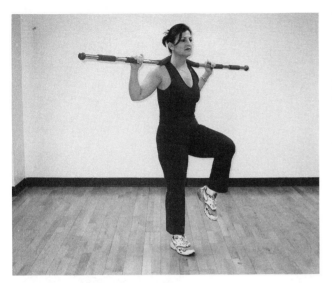

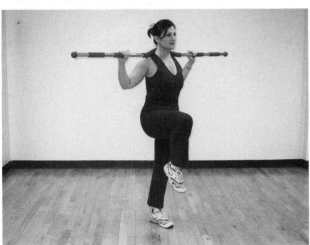

MARCH IN PLACE—30 to 50 reps

Rest the aerobic toning bar across your shoulders with feet shoulder width apart.

Raise left knee straight up to at least waist level. Keep back straight and abdominals contracted.

Lower left leg/foot to starting position. Repeat now with right leg and alternate legs for each repetition.

7. Fat Burner—5 minutes of biking or other aerobic piece, bouncing on trampoline, or walking.

8. Stand-ups.

STAND-UPS FROM THE FLOOR—5 TO 7 reps

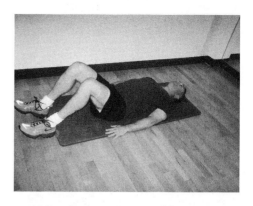

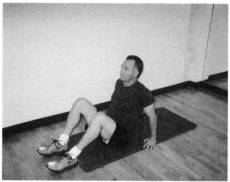

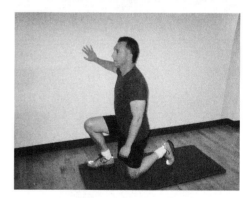

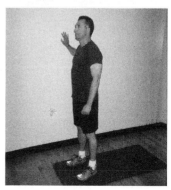

9. Upper Body Exercises: to be performed with the aerobic toning bar.

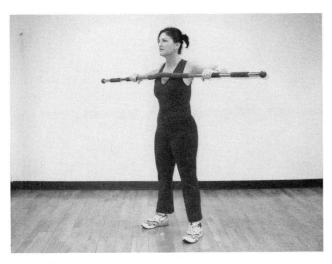

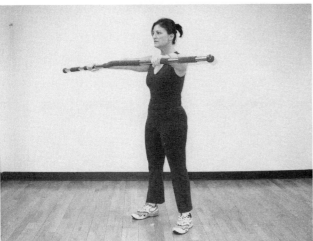

(a) PUSH-OUTS—25 reps

Keep back straight, knees slightly flexed, and feet shoulder width apart.

i. Grip bar, palms facing down, just past shoulder width. Raise bar up just above your chest line with elbows up and wrists firm.

ii. Extend arms straight out, holding bar above chest level, and exhale.

iii. While inhaling, bring bar back to starting position and repeat. Keep lower body aligned and still throughout entire exercise.

iv. Moderate speed throughout entire movement.

(b) KICK-BACKS—25 reps

Keep back straight, knees slightly flexed, and feet shoulder width apart.

i. Grip bar with arms fully extended at buttocks, palms facing outward.

ii. Keeping elbows stationary and wrists firm, lift bar away from your buttocks as far as possible while exhaling. Keeping arms straight, lower bar to buttocks while inhaling and repeat.

iii. Moderate speed throughout entire movement.

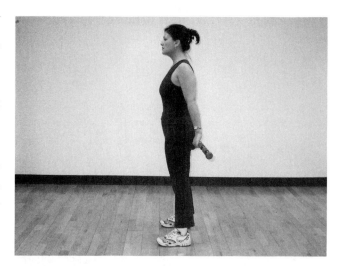

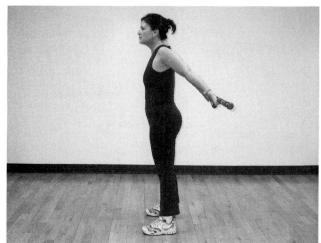

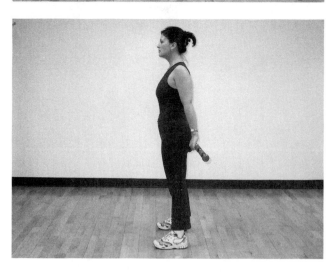

10. **Fat Burner**—5 minutes of biking or other aerobic piece, bouncing on trampoline, or walking.

11. **Cool down**—bike or walk for 3 minutes, nice and easy.

Workout #2—see page 110 for Off Day Routine prescription.

Plans for Losing 31–60 Pounds

Most Important Factor in Diet Plans

It is common for individuals in this weight category to sabotage their healthy eating plans. The end seems so far away, yet the extra weight may not seem so exorbitant. The weight loss may not be as fast as it was when you had more to lose. Individuals in this category often take two steps forward and one step back. It is important to figure out what is going on in your mind in order to break the cycle.

The best way to do this is to keep an eating diary. Record when, what, and why you eat. The why often turns out to be related to anxiety, depression, boredom, stress, et cetera. Once you know the whys, you can start to change those habits and start focusing on sufficiently fueling your body and not your emotions. Also, a simple rule to follow is this: Every time you overeat, the next day you must do an extra 30 minutes of aerobic exercise in order to "sweat out" those extra calories. Remember, there are consequences for overeating, so instead of beating yourself up for doing something bad, put it behind you and channel your energy in a more positive manner. With time, you will stop and say to yourself when you feel the urge to overeat, "Do I really need this?"

Helpful Tips for Successful Weight Reduction:

Keep a Food Journal—Write down what and when you eat and drink in a day and why: The journal will help you become aware of what you eat, will increase your control over eating, and will help you become aware of your eating patterns. Food becomes fattening when it is eaten for entertainment, comfort, or stress reduction.

Become Aware of Meal Timing: Eating earlier in the day prevents you from getting too hungry, losing control, and overeating in the evening.

Learn Your Calorie Budget: Know how much you can eat and still lose weight so you can be sure to fuel your body with an adequate amount of essential nutrients.

Eat Slowly: The brain needs about 20 minutes to receive the signal that you've eaten your fill. Practice by putting your fork down between bites and taking pauses throughout the meal.

Keep Away from Food Sources That Tempt You: Out of sight, out of mind, out of *mouth!* Hide high-calorie foods and keep healthy snacks readily available.

Taste Your Food: Calories should be tasted, not wasted. Do nothing else while eating and really savor your food.

Stick to Your Shopping List: Always bring a food list when grocery shopping and never shop while hungry!

Buy Individually-Wrapped Packages: Buy your favorite snack foods in individual serving sizes to avoid overeating and further temptation.

Set Realistic Goals: Weight loss greater than 1 percent of your body weight for over two weeks can be dangerous. You can lose muscle, including cardiac muscle. Aim to lose .5–2 pounds per week to ensure you are losing body fat.

Hidden Calorie Foods/Foods to Avoid

- Movie theater popcorn—large with butter contains 1,640 calories and 126 gm fat (73 gm saturated!)

- Prime rib—16 oz. contains 1,280 calories and 94 gm fat (52 gm saturated)

- Cheese—1 oz. contains 100 calories and 9 gm fat (6 gm saturated)

- Pizza—Domino's hand-tossed cheese (⅛ pie) contains 250 calories and 7 gm fat (4 gm saturated)

- General Tso's chicken—1,600 calories and 59 gm fat (11 gm saturated)

- Hamburgers—6-oz. burger on a bun contains 660 calories and 36 gm fat (17 gm saturated)

- Doughnuts—an old-fashioned cake doughnut contains 250 calories and 15 gm fat (3 gm saturated)

- Cinnamon rolls—670 calories and 34 gm fat (14 gm saturated)

- Croissants—5 oz. almond croissant contains 630 calories and 42 gm fat (18 gm saturated)

- French fries—large order contains 500 calories and 28 gm fat (13 gm saturated fat)

- Tortilla chips—typical basket (51 chips) contains 640 calories and 34 gm fat (6 gm saturated)

- Grilled-cheese sandwich—500 calories and 33 gm fat (17 gm saturated fat)

- Fettuccine alfredo—1,500 calories and 97 gm fat (48 gm saturated)

- Starbuck's white chocolate mocha (made with whole milk)—600 calories and 25 gm fat (15 gm saturated)

- Pancakes with syrup and margarine (3 pancakes with $1/4$ cup syrup and 1 tbsp. margarine)—770 calories and 22 gm fat (9 gm saturated)

*Please note: For those individuals who are vegetarian or have other special dietary needs, please log on to eatright.org or ediets.com to find a dietician near you.

Meal Plans for Losing 31–60 Pounds

Limited Approach

1600 CALORIES PER DAY

(221 GM CARBOHYDRATE, 80 GM PROTEIN, 44 GM FAT)

BREAKFAST *(500 calories, approx. 68 gm carbohydrate, 25 gm protein, 14 gm fat):*

1. (500 calories, 72 gm carb, 24 gm protein, 15 gm fat)

   2 $1/4$ cups whole grain cereal (unsweetened, ready-to-eat cereal)

   1 cup skim milk

   1 cup berries

   12 almonds

   1 hard-boiled egg

2. (500 calories, 66 gm carb, 33 gm protein, 15 gm fat)

   $1/2$ cup 1 percent cottage cheese

   1 cup berries

   1 cup melon

   12 almonds

   2 tbsp. Grape-Nuts

1 slice of whole grain bread

1 tsp. peanut butter

3. (500 calories, 67 gm carb, 26 gm protein, 13 gm fat)

    2 slices of whole grain bread

    1 tbsp. peanut butter

    1 apple

    12 oz. low-fat yogurt

4. (500 calories, 65 gm carb, 28 gm protein, 15 gm fat)

    2 poached eggs

    2 slices of whole grain bread

    3/4 cup plain low-fat yogurt

    1 1/2 cups melon

5. (500 calories, 63 gm carb, 23 gm protein, 15 gm fat)

1 1/2 cups cooked oatmeal

12 chopped walnut halves

1 chopped Red Delicious apple

1/2 cup low-fat cottage cheese

6. (500 calories, 65 gm carb, 25 gm protein, 10 gm fat)

    Omelet—1 whole egg and 2 egg whites + 1/2 oz. of low-fat cheese + 1/2 cup spinach + 1/2 cup chopped tomato

    2 slices of whole grain bread

    1 cup sliced strawberries

    1 sliced kiwi

7. (500 calories, 65 gm carb, 22 gm protein, 16 gm fat)

    2 slices of whole grain bread

    2 oz. cheese

    1/2 cup sliced tomato

    2 cups mixed melon

LUNCH *(500 calories, approx. 68 gm carbohydrate, 25 gm protein, 14 gm fat):*

1. (500 calories, 65 gm carb, 22 gm protein, 15 gm fat)

    2 slices of whole grain bread

    2 oz. white meat turkey

    1/4 avocado

    1/2 cup sliced tomato and lettuce

    1/2 cup unsweetened applesauce with 1/4 cup low-fat granola

2. (500 calories, 65 gm carb, 22 gm protein, 15 gm fat)

    1 whole wheat pita

    2 oz. chunk white tuna fish

3 tsps. mayonnaise

1/2 cup mixed shredded carrots, lettuce, and celery

24 cherries

3. (500 calories, 65 gm carb, 22 gm protein, 15 gm fat)

    2 oz. of cold chicken (cut up) mixed with 3 tsps. mayonnaise

    2 slices of rye bread

    1/2 cup sliced tomato and lettuce

    1 whole diced mango

4. (500 calories, 65 gm carb, 25 gm protein, 15 gm fat)

   Big Salad:

       2 cups mixed greens

       $1/2$ cup diced carrots

       $1/2$ cup diced bell peppers

       $1/3$ cup beans

   2 oz. grilled chicken

   4 chopped walnuts

   1 diced apple

   2 tbsps. vinaigrette salad dressing

   1 medium nectarine

5. (500 calories, 70 gm carb, 24 gm protein, 15 gm fat)

   2 oz. lean roast beef

   2 slices of rye bread

   1 tsp. mayonnaise

   $1/2$ cup sliced tomato and lettuce

   $1/2$ cup carrot sticks

   1 $1/2$ cups fresh pineapple topped with 6 slivered almonds

6. (500 calories, 60 gm carb, 28 gm protein, 15 gm fat)

   2 cups spinach

   1 oz. feta cheese

   1 oz. firm tofu

   $1/2$ cup water chestnuts

   $1/2$ cup snap peas

   $3/4$ cup mandarin oranges

   1 tbsp. reduced-fat ginger salad dressing

   10 whole grain crackers

7. (500 calories, 65 gm carb, 28 gm protein, 15 gm fat)

   2 slices of whole grain bread

   2 oz. white meat turkey

   1 oz. low-fat cheese

   2 tsps. mayonnaise

   $1/2$ cup sliced tomato and lettuce

   1 $1/2$ cups mixed fruit salad

DINNER *(600 calories, approx. 85 gm carbohydrate, 30 gm protein, 16 gm fat):*

1. (600 calories, 85 gm carb, 28 gm protein, 15 gm fat)

   2 oz. cooked chicken (no skin)

   1 cup brown rice

   1 cup green beans sautéed in 1 tsp. olive oil and 6 slivered almonds

   1 cup mixed greens with $1/2$ cup chopped tomatoes and $1/2$ cup chopped peppers

   1 tbsp. salad dressing

   1 medium apple

2. (600 calories, 85 gm carb, 26 gm protein, 16 gm fat)

   2 oz. lean cooked roast beef

   $2/3$ cup brown rice

   $1/2$ cup carrots

   $1/2$ cup cauliflower

   2 tsps. olive oil

   1 whole grain dinner roll

   1 orange

3. (600 calories, 83 gm carb, 29 gm protein, 16 gm fat)

   2 oz. broiled salmon

   1 large sweet potato

   1 cup sautéed spinach with 2 tsps. olive oil

   1 cup sliced tomato

   1 1/2 cups diced melon

4. (600 calories, 85 gm carb, 30 gm protein, 16 gm fat)

   2 oz. sautéed shrimp in 2 tsps. olive oil

   1 1/2 cups whole wheat pasta

   1/2 cup jarred tomato sauce

   1/2 cup artichoke hearts

   1/2 cup spinach

   1 1/4 cups sliced strawberries

   1 sliced fresh peach

5. (600 calories, 80 gm carb, 32 gm protein, 16 gm fat)

   3 oz. baked cod

   1/3 cup cooked whole wheat couscous

   2 cups baked winter squash

   1 cup mixed greens (kale, collard, and mustard) sautéed in 3 tsps. olive oil

   2 cups cubed papaya

6. (600 calories, 85 gm carb, 27 gm protein, 16 gm fat)

   2 oz. flank steak

   1 cup whole wheat couscous

   2 cups roasted broccoli and cauliflower with 2 tsps. olive oil

   1 1/2 cups raspberries

7. (500 calories, 83 gm carb, 27 gm protein, 16 gm fat)

   2 oz. barbecued chicken

   1 medium corn on the cob

   1 cup baked beans

   1 1/2 cups cucumber and tomato salad tossed with 2 tbsps. olive oil–based dressing

   1/2 cup cubed watermelon

Dynamic Approach
2000 CALORIES PER DAY
(274 GM CARBOHYDRATE, 98 GM PROTEIN, 56 GM FAT)

BREAKFAST (600 calories, approx. 82 gm carbohydrate, 30 gm protein, 16 gm fat):

1. (600 calories, 82 gm carb, 28 gm protein, 15 gm fat)

   2 1/4 cups whole grain cereal (unsweetened, ready-to-eat cereal)

   1 1/2 cups skim milk

   1 1/4 cups berries

   12 almonds

   1 hard-boiled egg

2. (600 calories, 85 gm carb, 36 gm protein, 17 gm fat)

   1/2 cup 1 percent cottage cheese

1 cup berries

1 cup melon

1/3 cup Grape-Nuts

12 almonds

1 slice of whole grain bread

2 tsps. peanut butter

3. (600 calories, 82 gm carb, 29 gm protein, 15 gm fat)

2 slices of whole grain bread

1 tbsp. peanut butter

1 apple

12 oz. low-fat yogurt

1/2 cup low-fat granola

4. (600 calories, 80 gm carb, 28 gm protein, 15 gm fat)

2 poached eggs

2 slices of whole grain bread

3/4 cup plain low-fat yogurt

1 1/2 cups melon

1 cup mixed berries

5. (600 calories, 78 gm carb, 33 gm protein, 15 gm fat)

2 cups cooked oatmeal

12 chopped walnut halves

1 chopped Red Delicious apple

3/4 cup low-fat cottage cheese

6. (600 calories, 80 gm carb, 27 gm protein, 15 gm fat)

Omelet—2 whole eggs + 1/2 oz. of low-fat cheese + 1/2 cup spinach + 1/2 cup chopped tomato

2 slices of whole grain bread

1 cup sliced strawberries

1 sliced kiwi

1 cup cubed melon

7. (600 calories, 84 gm carb, 30 gm protein, 16 gm fat)

2 slices of whole grain bread

2 oz. cheese

1/2 cup sliced tomato

2 1/2 cups mixed melon

1 cup skim milk

LUNCH *(600 calories, approx. 82 gm carbohydrate, 30 gm protein, 16 gm fat):*

1. 600 calories, 80 gm carb, 29 gm protein, 15 gm fat)

2 slices of whole grain bread

3 oz. white meat turkey

1/4 avocado

1/2 cup sliced tomato and lettuce

1 cup unsweetened applesauce with 1/4 cup low-fat granola

2. (600 calories, 80 gm carb, 29 gm protein, 15 gm fat)

1 whole wheat pita

3 oz. chunk white tuna fish

3 tsps. mayonnaise

1/2 cup mixed shredded carrots, lettuce, and celery

36 cherries

3. (600 calories, 80 gm carb, 29 gm protein, 15 gm fat)

   3 oz. of cold chicken (cut up) mixed with 3 tsps. mayonnaise

   2 slices of rye bread

   1/2 cup sliced tomato and lettuce

   1 whole diced mango

   1 cup raspberries

4. (600 calories, 80 gm carb, 35 gm protein, 15 gm fat)

   Big Salad:

       2 cups mixed greens

       1/2 cup diced carrots

       1/2 cup diced bell peppers

       1/3 cup beans

       3 oz. grilled chicken

       4 chopped walnuts

       1 diced apple

       2 tbsps. vinaigrette salad dressing

   1 medium nectarine

   six-inch whole wheat pita

5. (600 calories, 85 gm carb, 31 gm protein, 15 gm fat)

   3 oz. lean roast beef

   2 slices of rye bread

   1 tsp. mayonnaise

   1/2 cup sliced tomato and lettuce

   1/2 cup carrot sticks

   1 1/2 cups fresh pineapple + 1 cup diced papaya topped with 6 slivered almonds

6. (600 calories, 80 gm carb, 30 gm protein, 15 gm fat)

   3 cups spinach

   1 oz. feta cheese

   1 oz. firm tofu

   1/2 cup water chestnuts

   1/2 cup snap peas

   1 1/2 cups mandarin oranges

   1 tbsp. reduced-fat ginger salad dressing

   10 whole grain crackers

7. (600 calories, 80 gm carb, 31 gm protein, 15 gm fat)

   2 slices of whole grain bread

   2 oz. white meat turkey

   1 oz. low-fat cheese

   2 tsps. mayonnaise

   1/2 cup sliced tomato and lettuce

   1 1/2 cups mixed fruit salad

   3 whole wheat graham crackers

SNACK *(200 calories, approx. 27 gm carbohydrate, 10 gm protein, 6 gm fat):*

1. (200 calories, 27 gm carb, 8 gm protein, 5 gm fat)

   1 cup plain nonfat yogurt

   3/4 cup fresh blackberries

   6 chopped almonds

2. (200 calories, 27 gm carb, 8 gm protein, 5 gm fat)

   1 medium apple

   2 tsps. peanut butter

   1 cup skim milk

3. (200 calories, 30 gm carb, 7 gm protein, 7 gm fat)

   1 whole grain English muffin

   1 oz. Swiss cheese

4. (200 calories, 27 gm carb, 8 gm protein, 5 gm fat)

   Peanut-butter-and-jelly smoothie: Blend 1 cup skim milk + 1 1/4 cups fresh or frozen strawberries + 2 tsps. peanut butter

5. (200 calories, 27 gm carb, 8 gm protein, 5 gm fat)

   six-inch whole wheat pita

   1 sliced apple

   2 tsps. peanut butter

6. (200 calories, 27 gm carb, 8 gm protein, 5 gm fat)

   1 slice whole wheat raisin bread topped with 1 sliced kiwi and 1/4 cup ricotta cheese

7. (200 calories, 27 gm carb, 8 gm protein, 5 gm fat)

   1/2 six-inch whole wheat pita

   1/3 cup hummus

   1/2 cup carrot sticks

DINNER *(600 calories, approx. 82 gm carbohydrate, 30 gm protein, 16 gm fat):*

1. (600 calories, 85 gm carb, 28 gm protein, 15 gm fat)

   2 oz. cooked chicken (no skin)

   1 cup brown rice

   1 cup green beans sautéed in 1 tsp. olive oil and 6 slivered almonds

   1 cup mixed greens with 1/2 cup chopped tomatoes and 1/2 cup chopped peppers

   1 tbsp. salad dressing

   1 medium apple

2. (600 calories, 85 gm carb, 26 gm protein, 16 gm fat)

   2 oz. lean cooked roast beef

   2/3 cup brown rice

   1/2 cup carrots

   1/2 cup cauliflower

   2 tsps. olive oil

   1 whole grain dinner roll

   1 orange

3. (600 calories, 83 gm carb, 29 gm protein, 16 gm fat)

   2 oz. broiled salmon

   1 large sweet potato

   1 cup sautéed spinach with 2 tsps. olive oil

   1 cup sliced tomato

   1 1/2 cups diced melon

4. (600 calories, 85 gm carb, 30 gm protein, 16 gm fat)

   2 oz. sautéed shrimp in 2 tsps. olive oil

   1 1/2 cups whole wheat pasta

   1/2 cup jarred tomato sauce

   1/2 cup artichoke hearts

   1/2 cup spinach

   1 1/4 cups sliced strawberries

   1 sliced fresh peach

5. (600 calories, 80 gm carb, 32 gm protein, 16 gm fat)

    3 oz. baked cod

    $^1/_3$ cup cooked whole wheat couscous

    2 cups baked winter squash

    1 cup mixed greens (kale, collard, and mustard) sautéed in 3 tsps. olive oil

    2 cups cubed papaya

6. (600 calories, 85 gm carb, 27 gm protein, 16 gm fat)

    2 oz. flank steak

    1 cup whole wheat couscous

    2 cups roasted broccoli and cauliflower with 2 tsps. olive oil

    1 $^1/_2$ cups raspberries

7. (500 calories, 83 gm carb, 27 gm protein, 16 gm fat)

    2 oz. barbecued chicken

    1 medium corn on the cob

    1 cup baked beans

    1 $^1/_2$ cups cucumber and tomato salad tossed with 2 tbsps. olive oil–based dressing

    $^1/_2$ cup cubed watermelon

Balanced Approach
1800 CALORIES PER DAY
(247 GM CARBOHYDRATE, 90 GM PROTEIN, 50 GM FAT)

BREAKFAST *(500 calories, approx. 68 gm carbohydrate, 25 gm protein, 14 gm fat):*

1. (500 calories, 72 gm carb, 24 gm protein, 15 gm fat)

    2 $^1/_4$ cups whole grain cereal (unsweetened, ready-to-eat cereal)

    1 cup skim milk

    1 cup berries

    12 almonds

    1 hard-boiled egg

2. (500 calories, 66 gm carb, 33 gm protein, 15 gm fat)

    $^1/_2$ cup 1 percent cottage cheese

    1 cup berries

    1 cup melon

    12 almonds

    2 tbsp. Grape-Nuts

    1 slice of whole grain bread

3. (500 calories, 67 gm carb, 26 gm protein, 13 gm fat)

    2 slices of whole grain bread

    1 tbsp. peanut butter

    1 apple

    12 oz. low-fat yogurt

4. (500 calories, 65 gm carb, 28 gm protein, 15 gm fat)

    2 poached eggs

    2 slices of whole grain bread

    $^3/_4$ cup plain low-fat yogurt

    1 $^1/_2$ cups melon

5. (500 calories, 63 gm carb, 23 gm protein, 15 gm fat)

    1 $^1/_2$ cups cooked oatmeal

12 chopped walnut halves

1 chopped Red Delicious apple

1/2 cup low-fat cottage cheese

6. (500 calories, 65 gm carb, 25 gm protein, 10 gm fat)

Omelet—1 whole egg and 2 egg whites + 1/2 oz. low-fat cheese + 1/2 cup spinach + 1/2 cup chopped tomato

2 slices of whole grain bread

1 cup sliced strawberries

1 sliced kiwi

7. (500 calories, 65 gm carb, 22 gm protein, 16 gm fat)

2 slices of whole grain bread

2 oz. cheese

1/2 cup sliced tomato

2 cups mixed melon

LUNCH *(500 calories, approx. 68 gm carbohydrate, 25 gm protein, 14 gm fat):*

1. (500 calories, 65 gm carb, 22 gm protein, 15 gm fat)

2 slices of whole grain bread

2 oz. white meat turkey

1/4 avocado

1/2 cup sliced tomato and lettuce

1/2 cup unsweetened applesauce with 1/4 cup low-fat granola

2. (500 calories, 65 gm carb, 22 gm protein, 15 gm fat)

1 whole wheat pita

2 oz. chunk white tuna fish

3 tsps. mayonnaise

1/2 cup mixed shredded carrots, lettuce, and celery

24 cherries

3. (500 calories, 65 gm carb, 22 gm protein, 15 gm fat)

2 oz. of cold chicken (cut up) mixed with 3 tsps. mayonnaise

2 slices of rye bread

1/2 cup sliced tomato and lettuce

1 whole diced mango

4. (500 calories, 65 gm carb, 25 gm protein, 15 gm fat)

Big Salad:

2 cups mixed greens

1/2 cup diced carrots

1/2 cup diced bell peppers

1/3 cup beans

2 oz. grilled chicken

4 chopped walnuts

1 diced apple

2 tbsps. vinaigrette salad dressing

1 medium nectarine

5. (500 calories, 70 gm carb, 24 gm protein, 15 gm fat)

2 oz. lean roast beef

2 slices of rye bread

1 tsp. mayonnaise

1/2 cup sliced tomato and lettuce

1/2 cup carrot sticks

1 1/2 cups fresh pineapple topped with 6 slivered almonds

6. (500 calories, 60 gm carb, 28 gm protein, 15 gm fat)

2 cups spinach

1 oz. feta cheese

1 oz. firm tofu

1/2 cup water chestnuts

1/2 cup snap peas

3/4 cup mandarin oranges

1 tbsp. reduced-fat ginger salad dressing

10 whole grain crackers

7. (500 calories, 65 gm carb, 28 gm protein, 15 gm fat)

2 slices of whole grain bread

2 oz. white meat turkey

1 oz. low-fat cheese

2 tsps. mayonnaise

1/2 cup sliced tomato and lettuce

1 1/2 cups mixed fruit salad

SNACK *(200 calories, approx. 27 gm carbohydrate, 10 gm protein, 6 gm fat):*

1. (200 calories, 27 gm carb, 8 gm protein, 5 gm fat)

1 cup plain nonfat yogurt

3/4 cup fresh blackberries

6 chopped almonds

2. (200 calories, 27 gm carb, 8 gm protein, 5 gm fat)

1 medium apple

2 tsps. peanut butter

1 cup skim milk

3. (200 calories, 30 gm carb, 7 gm protein, 7 gm fat)

1 whole grain English muffin

1 oz. Swiss cheese

4. (200 calories, 27 gm carb, 8 gm protein, 5 gm fat)

Peanut-butter-and-jelly smoothie:

Blend 1 cup skim milk + 1 1/4 cups fresh or frozen strawberries + 2 tsps. peanut butter

5. (200 calories, 27 gm carb, 8 gm protein, 5 gm fat)

six-inch whole wheat pita

1 sliced apple

2 tsps. peanut butter

6. (200 calories, 27 gm carb, 8 gm protein, 5 gm fat)

1 slice whole wheat raisin bread topped with 1 sliced kiwi and 1/4 cup ricotta cheese

7. (200 calories, 27 gm carb, 8 gm protein, 5 gm fat)

1/2 six-inch whole wheat pita

1/3 cup hummus

1/2 cup carrot sticks

DINNER *(600 calories, approx. 85 gm carbohydrate, 30 gm protein, 16 gm fat):*

1. **(600 calories, 85 gm carb, 28 gm protein, 15 gm fat)**

   2 oz. cooked chicken (no skin)

   1 cup brown rice

   1 cup green beans sautéed in 1 tsp. olive oil and 6 slivered almonds

   1 cup mixed greens with 1/2 cup chopped tomatoes and 1/2 cup chopped peppers

   1 tbsp. salad dressing

   1 medium apple

2. **(600 calories, 85 gm carb, 26 gm protein, 16 gm fat)**

   2 oz. lean cooked roast beef

   2/3 cup brown rice

   1/2 cup carrots

   1/2 cup cauliflower

   2 tsps. olive oil

   1 whole grain dinner roll

   1 orange

3. **(600 calories, 83 gm carb, 29 gm protein, 16 gm fat)**

   2 oz. broiled salmon

   1 large sweet potato

   1 cup sautéed spinach with 2 tsps. olive oil

   1 cup sliced tomato

   1 1/2 cups diced melon

4. **(600 calories, 85 gm carb, 30 gm protein, 16 gm fat)**

   2 oz. sautéed shrimp in 2 tsps. olive oil

   1 1/2 cups whole wheat pasta

   1/2 cup jarred tomato sauce

   1/2 cup artichoke hearts

   1/2 cup spinach

   1 1/4 cups sliced strawberries

   1 sliced fresh peach

5. **(600 calories, 80 gm carb, 32 gm protein, 16 gm fat)**

   3 oz. baked cod

   1/3 cup cooked whole wheat couscous

   2 cups baked winter squash

   1 cup mixed greens (kale, collard, and mustard) sautéed in 3 tsps. olive oil

   2 cups cubed papaya

6. **(600 calories, 85 gm carb, 27 gm protein, 16 gm fat)**

   2 oz. flank steak

   1 cup whole wheat couscous

   2 cups roasted broccoli and cauliflower with 2 tsps. olive oil

   1 1/2 cups raspberries

7. **(500 calories, 83 gm carb, 27 gm protein, 16 gm fat)**

   2 oz. barbecued chicken

   1 medium corn on the cob

   1 cup baked beans

   1 1/2 cups cucumber and tomato salad tossed with 2 tbsps. olive oil–based dressing

   1/2 cup cubed watermelon

Additional Foods to Choose as Between Meal Snacks

LOW-CALORIE

Fresh fruit

Fresh vegetables (can dip them in 2 tbsps. hummus, salsa, or homemade low-fat dip)

Low-fat yogurt

Low-fat cottage cheese

Hot-air-popped popcorn

MEDIUM-CALORIE

$1/4$ cup dry-roasted nuts (need to limit portions)

1 tbsp. nut butter on a slice of whole wheat bread

1 tbsp. nut butter on a medium apple

2 tsps. peanut butter + 2 graham crackers + 2 tsps. jam

1 oz. of reduced-fat cheese with 10 whole grain crackers

1 slice of reduced-fat cheese melted over tomato on whole grain bread

Nonfat Greek yogurt with 1 cup of berries and 2 tbsps. chopped nuts

$1/4$ cup dry-roasted mixed nuts (almonds, pumpkinseeds, walnuts)

$1/2$ whole wheat English muffin + 1 slice low-fat mozzarella cheese + 1 tbsp. marinara sauce

1 medium orange diced into 1 serving of oatmeal + 2 walnut halves

FOR SWEET CRAVINGS

Fresh watermelon

Fresh berries

Sugar-free Jell-O

Fat-free/sugar-free fudge pop

Sugar-free Popsicle

FOR SAVORY CRAVINGS

Fresh vegetables dipped in salsa

Hot-air-popped popcorn

Exercise Prescription for Losing 31–60 Pounds

Most Important Factor

The most important factors that will ensure weight loss for you are two things: First, try to work out a minimum of 3 days a week performing your full-body routine; and second, decrease your caloric intake, especially on the days you don't work out or aren't very active. Just remember, each day that you don't eat sensibly, you need to counter that with an extra day of working out to ensure and maintain long-term weight loss.

Fitness Equipment Needed

1. **Choose One:** Recumbent or upright stationary bike, treadmill, elliptical machine or cross trainer or, if no access to any equipment, walk/jog instead

2. Firm exercise mat

3. A lightweight (2–4 lb.) collapsible aerobic toning bar for both men and women

4. A 10–15 lb. weighted bar for men

5. Trampoline (optional)

6. A lightweight speed or beaded jump rope

   (See pages 140–141 for photos of fitness equipment needed.)

While jumping rope, make sure you jump on a surface that has some give to it, such as a wooden floor, short grass, a rubberized track or tennis court, or the like. *Do not* jump on asphalt or cement. If you don't have access to this type of surface and/or need help in improving your jump rope skills, log onto *www.exude.com* to view Jump Rope Mat and Jumping Rope Videos.

Please Note: All of the following exercise regimens can be performed at home, at the gym, or even while traveling.

Exercise Regimen
Frequency—2, 3, 4, or 5 days per week
Duration—50 to 60 minutes, depending upon your current level of fitness

**Before starting this or any exercise regimen, get your doctor's approval.*

Workout #1
Full-Body Routine—2 to 3 days per week, every other day, Mondays, Wednesdays, and Fridays or Tuesdays, Thursdays, and Saturdays.

"Reps" = Repetitions; the number of times you actually perform the exercise.

1. **Warm-up**—bike, brisk walk, light jog, or elliptical or cross trainer for 30 minutes with high speed, 85 + RPMs with low resistance, or walk at 3.5 + MPH or jog at 5.0 + MPH, with no incline.

   Please Note: If you are unable to perform 30 continuous minutes of aerobic exercise, take a break for a minute or so, then resume until you've completed 30 minutes.

2. **Stretch**—4 minutes.

3. **Fat Burner**—(a) jump rope or trampoline for 1 minute, then (b) 3 minutes of biking, walking, jogging, or aerobic piece of your choice, with moderate intensity. (If unable to jump rope or use trampoline, do 4 minutes of aerobic of your choice.)

4. **Legs/Hips**—(a) standing knee to opposite chest: 20 to 30 reps; (b) L kicks: 20 to 30 reps; (c) march in place on toes: 50 to 60 reps.

5. **Jumping Jacks**—40 to 50 reps.

6. **Upper Body Exercises**—with aerobic toning bar for women and a 10-15 lb weighted bar for men: (a) push-outs: 35 reps; (b) front press: 35 reps; (c) upright rows: 35 reps; (d) curls: 35 reps; (e) kick-backs: 35 reps.

7. **Fat Burner**—(a) jump rope or trampoline for 1 minute, then (b) 3 minutes of biking, walking, jogging, or aerobic piece of your choice, with moderate intensity. (If unable to jump rope or use trampoline, do 4 minutes of aerobic of your choice.)

8. **Abdominals/Legs**—(a) sit-ups: 30 to 40 reps; (b) leg-outs: 20 reps, rest 10 seconds, then repeat 20 reps; (c) alternates: 20 reps, then rest 10 seconds, then repeat 20 reps; (d) v-scissors (women only): 20 reps, then rest 10 seconds, then repeat 20 reps; (e) knees to chest: 20 reps; (f) elbows to knees: 20 reps.

9. **Fat Burner**—(a) Jump rope or bounce on trampoline for 1 minute, then (b) 3 minutes of biking, walking, jogging, or aerobic piece of your choice, with moderate intensity. (If unable to jump rope or use trampoline, do 4 minutes of aerobic of your choice.)

10. **Jumping Jacks**—40 to 50 reps.

11. **Cooldown**—3 minutes of biking or walking leisurely.

If you need a break at any time during your exercise regimen, you can simply get on a stationary bike or any other piece of aerobic equipment or walk for 1–3 minutes to allow your heart rate to come down safely before you resume. Also, if you want to pay more attention to either your upper body, midsection, or lower body, you can either perform more repetitions or do an extra set of exercises that target that region.

Based upon your time allotment and level of fitness, you can either cool down or perform another set of upper body exercises, #6, and another set of abdominals/legs, #8, and then cool down afterward. If you can perform more repetitions with any exercise, please go ahead and do so. If not, keep track of how many repetitions you do for all of your exercises, and as you increase your fitness level you will then be able to comfortably increase the number of repetitions you perform with any and all exercises. Try to add 1–2 repetitions for each exercise every two to three weeks, working up to 50–60 repetitions for each exercise. Also, work up to 4 full minutes of rope jumping for each Fat Burner.

1. Aerobic Equipment

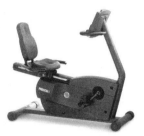

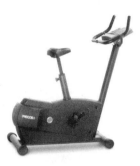

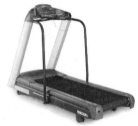

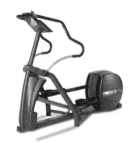

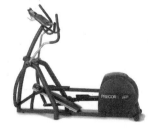

Workout #2 (Optional, depending upon which approach you choose: Balanced or Dynamic)

Off Day Routine—2 to 3 days per week on days in between Full-Body Routines.

1. Aerobic exercise of your choice for 40 minutes with moderate intensity.

2. Stretch—4 minutes.

3. Jumping jacks—40 to 50 reps.

4. Abdominals/Legs—(a) sit-ups: 40 reps, (b) leg-outs: 25 reps; (c) v-scissors: 25 reps; (d) alternates: 40 reps; (e) elbows to knees: 20 reps; (f) knees to elbows: 20 reps.

5. Jumping jacks—40 to 50 reps.

6. Cooldown—3 minutes of leisurely biking or walking.

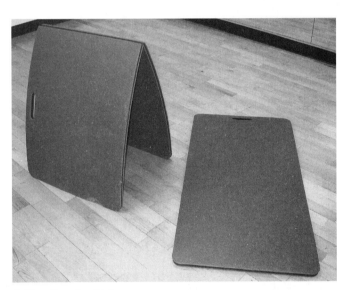

2. Firm Exercise Mat

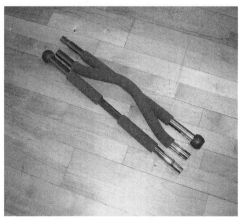
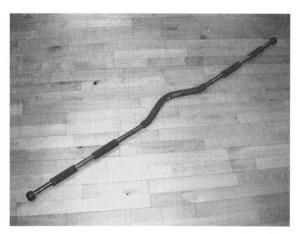

3. Collapsible Aerobic Toning Bar   Unassembled   Assembled

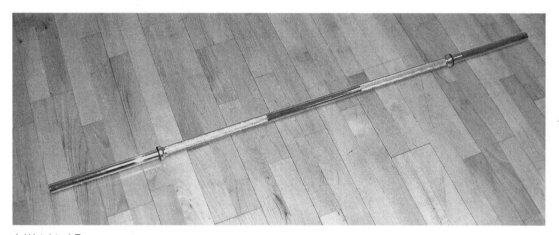

4. Weighted Bar

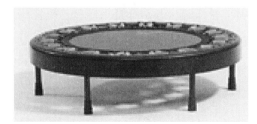

5. Trampoline

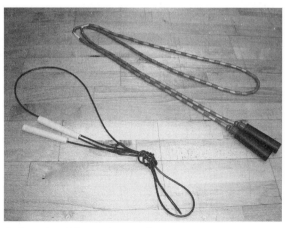

6. Speed and Beaded Jump Rope

Workout #1—Full-Body Routine

1. Warm-up—30 minutes

2. Stretch—hold each stretch for 30–60 seconds.

ARM CIRCLES

With arms outstretched, slowly circle your arms backward for 5 revolutions and then forward for 5 revolutions.

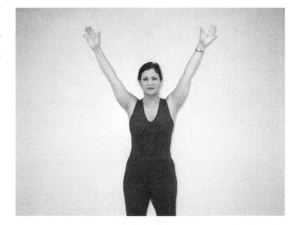

TRICEPS

With arms overhead, gently pull the left elbow behind your head with your right hand. Hold when you reach a comfortable stretch in the rear shoulder and upper back. Switch arms and repeat.

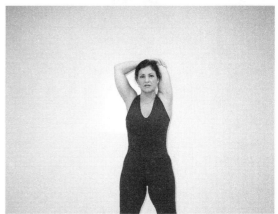

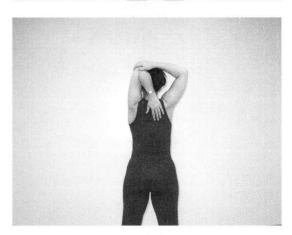

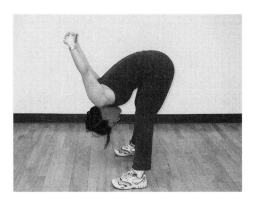

SHOULDERS, CHEST, AND HAMSTRINGS

Grasp hands behind your back, with palms facing each other. Slightly bend your knees and lift arms up as you bend forward at the waist. Hold when you feel a comfortable stretch in the shoulders, chest, and hamstrings.

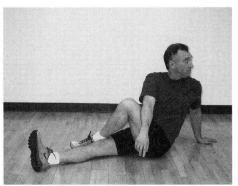

SPINAL TWIST

Keeping the right leg straight, left arm behind for support, cross left leg over and place foot outside the right knee. With the right hand or elbow on the left knee, slowly twist and look over your left shoulder while simultaneously pulling the knee in the opposite direction; hold. You will feel pressure in the hip, side, and upper back. Repeat on opposite side.

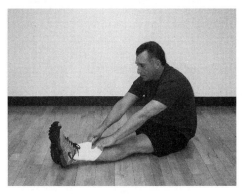

HAMSTRINGS

With legs straight, ankles flexed, bend forward from the hips and reach out toward your toes and, based on your flexibility, grab on to either your socks, shoelaces, or toes while holding the stretch. You will feel tension just behind the knees, in the upper calves, and in the lower back area. If possible, you should also perform this stretch with legs apart, using the preceding instructions.

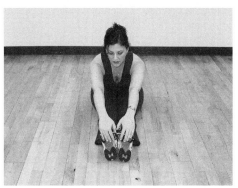

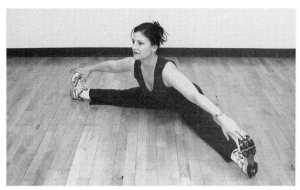

GROIN

In sitting position, pull the soles of your feet together and grab hold of your ankles. Gently pull heels toward the groin area. Let your knees relax toward the floor, and gently press your elbows down on your knees to increase the stretch.

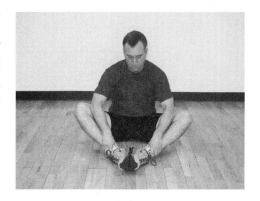

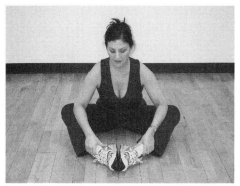

QUADRICEPS

Lie down on your left side. Bend your right leg back and grab your right ankle with your right hand. Gently pull your right leg back toward your buttocks. Hold the position when you feel a comfortable stretch in front of your right thigh. Release slowly and roll over to your left side and repeat.

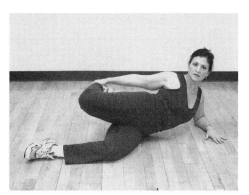

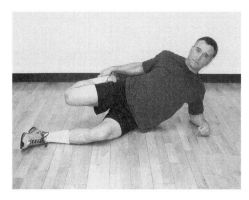

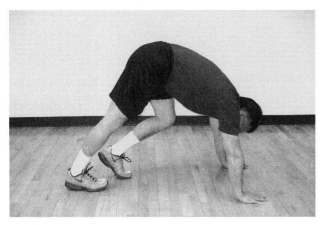

CALVES #1

With hands and knees on all fours, straighten your body into a V position. With both feet together, bend your left knee and press your right heel toward the ground, stretching your right calf. Repeat on other side.

OR

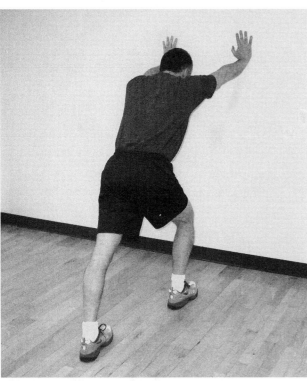

CALVES #2

Stand a little farther than arms' length away from a wall or solid support; lean on it with hands placed shoulder distance away. Bring one foot forward, knee bent, while keeping the back leg straight, heel pressing into the floor. Lean toward wall while holding stretch. Switch legs and repeat.

3. **Fat Burner**—(a) jump rope or bounce on trampoline for 1 minute, then (b) 3 minutes of biking, walking, jogging, or aerobic piece of your choice, with moderate intensity. (If unable to jump rope or use trampoline, do 4 minutes of aerobic of your choice.)

(a) JUMPING ROPE–1 MINUTE

How to Jump Rope:

i. Practice swinging rope overhead without jumping, forming a loop.

ii. Move forearms in time with feet.

iii. Jump just high enough for rope to pass under feet (one inch off the ground). Jump with both feet at once. (Jumping higher than one inch will create unnecessary stress on the legs, increasing the potential for injury.)

iv. Rope should hit the ground about one foot in front of feet with each revolution.

v. Caution: Avoid double jumping. Your workout will not be as effective! After each jump the rope should pass under your feet.

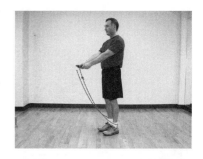
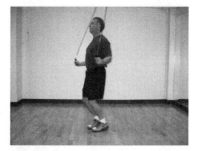
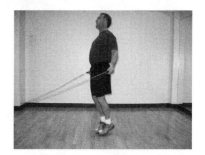
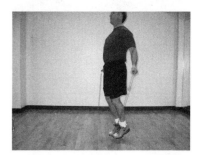
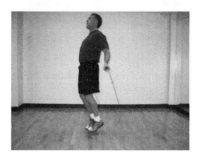

(b) 3 MINUTES OF AEROBIC EXERCISE

4. Legs/Hips.

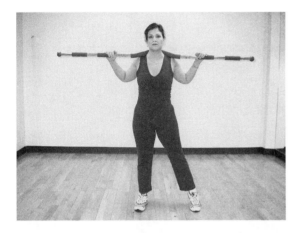

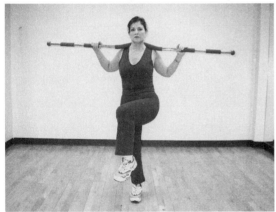

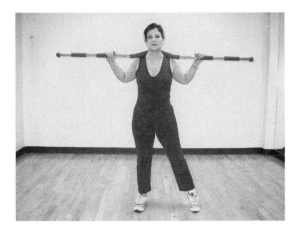

(a) STANDING KNEE TO OPPOSITE CHEST—20 to 30 reps

Rest the aerobic toning Bar on your neck across your shoulders, with feet shoulder width apart.

i.   Transfer all weight to your right leg.

ii. Raise left knee up toward your right chest to at least waist-chest level.

iii. Lower left foot to starting position, touching the ground while keeping your weight on your right leg throughout the movement. Switch legs and repeat.

iv. Try to keep aerobic bar straight across back/shoulders while performing exercise.

(b) L KICKS—20 to 30 reps

Hold the aerobic toning bar upright with your right hand and place your left hand on your waist.

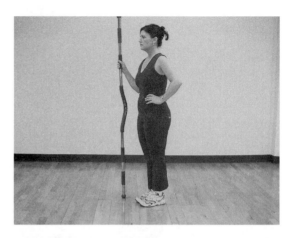

i.   Start by raising your left leg and trying to get it to waist level, keeping it as straight as possible, pointing your toe without leaning your weight on the bar.

ii. Then return to starting position, lightly touching the ground.

iii. Raise the left leg out to the side as high as possible, keeping it as straight as possible, pointing your toe without leaning your weight on the bar.

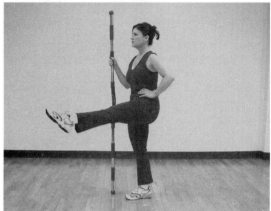

iv. Return to starting position and repeat.

v.   After you have completed all of your repetitions with your left leg, switch legs and repeat with your right leg while holding the aerobic toning bar with your left hand.

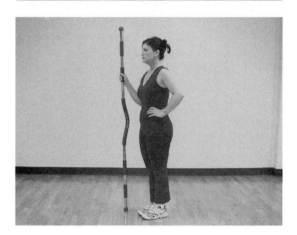

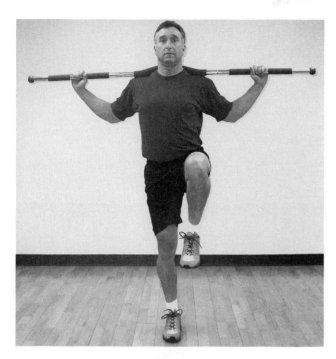

(c) MARCH IN PLACE ON TOES—75 reps

i. Rest the aerobic toning bar across your shoulders with feet about shoulder width apart and raise up to your toes.

ii. Raise left knee straight up to at least waist level toward your chest. Keep back straight and abdominals contracted.

iii. Lower left leg to starting position to toes, making sure that your heels do not touch ground throughout entire movement.

iv. Alternate legs through entire exercise.

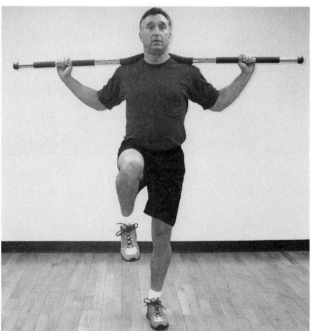

5. Jumping jacks 40 to 50 reps

Start with arms extended fully over head and legs apart. While exhaling, simultaneously bring arms down and touch hands on each side of the outside of thighs while shuffling feet together, barely lifting feet off the ground. Inhale as you return to starting position and repeat, keeping arms as straight as possible during entire movement.

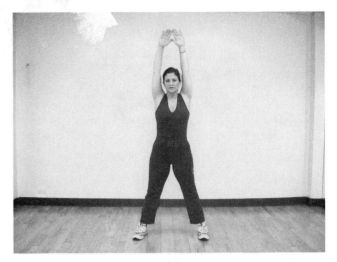

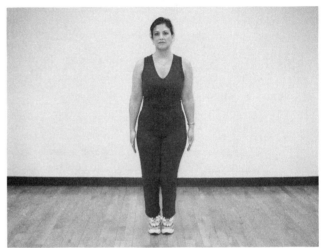

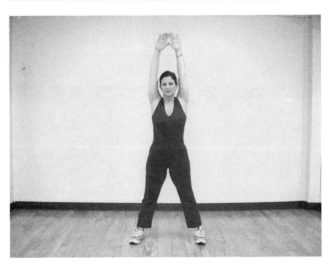

6. Upper Body Exercises—with aerobic toning bar for women and a weighted bar for men.

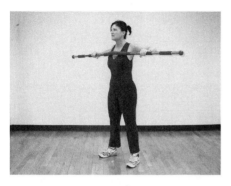

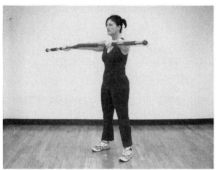

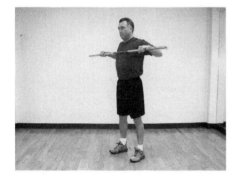

(a) PUSH-OUTS—35 reps

Keep back straight, knees slightly flexed, and feet shoulder width apart.

i. Grip bar, palms facing down, just past shoulder width. Raise bar up just above your chest line with elbows up and wrists firm.
ii. Extend arms straight out, holding bar above chest level, and exhale.
iii. While inhaling, bring bar back to starting position and repeat. Keep lower body aligned and still throughout entire exercise.
iv. Moderate speed throughout entire movement.

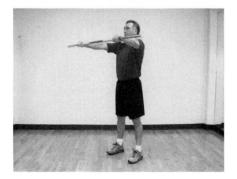

(b) FRONT PRESS—35 reps

Keep back straight, knees slightly flexed, and feet shoulder width apart.

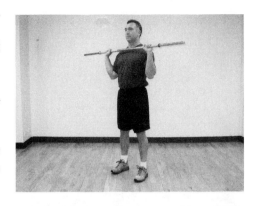

i.   Grip bar just past shoulder width and rest bar across top of chest.

ii. Fully extend arms upward and raise bar straight up while exhaling. Bend arms and slowly return bar to top of chest while inhaling and repeat.

iii. Moderate speed throughout entire movement.

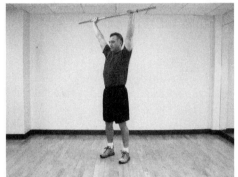

(c) UPRIGHT ROWS—35 reps

Keep back straight, knees slightly flexed, and feet shoulder width apart.

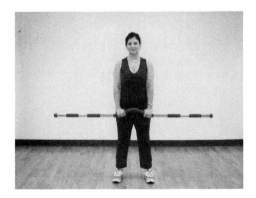

i.   Grip bar, palms facing down, six to eight inches apart. Hold bar with arms fully extended at front of thighs.

ii. Slowly raise bar up to chin, keeping elbows at or above bar level while exhaling. Return to starting position while inhaling and repeat.

iii. Moderate speed throughout entire movement.

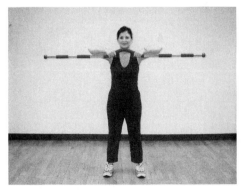

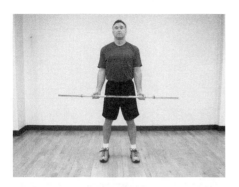

(d) CURLS—35 reps

Keep back straight, knees slightly flexed, and feet shoulder width apart.

i. Grip bar, palms facing up and shoulder width apart. Hold bar with arms fully extended at front of thighs.

ii. Keeping elbows stationary and wrists firm, curl bar up to chest while exhaling. Slowly extend arms and return bar to start position while inhaling and repeat.

iii. Moderate speed throughout entire movement.

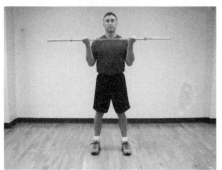

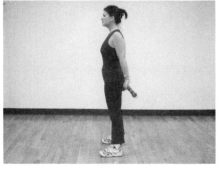

(e) KICK-BACKS—35 reps

Keep back straight, knees slightly flexed, and feet shoulder width apart.

i. Grip bar with arms fully extended at buttocks, palms facing outward about shoulder width apart.

ii. Keeping elbows stationary and wrists firm, lift bar away from your buttocks as far as possible while exhaling. Keeping arms straight, lower bar to buttocks while inhaling and repeat.

iii. Moderate speed throughout entire movement.

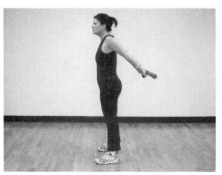

7. **Fat Burner**—(a) jump rope or bounce on trampoline for 1 minute, then (b) 3 minutes of biking, walking, jogging, or aerobic piece of your choice, with moderate intensity. (If unable to jump rope or use trampoline, do 4 minutes of aerobic of your choice.)

(a) JUMP ROPE–1 minute

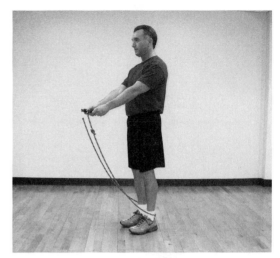

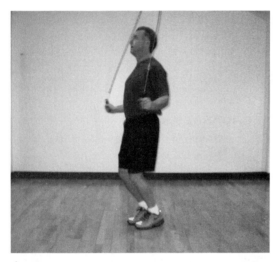

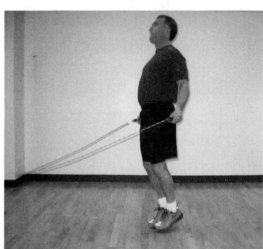

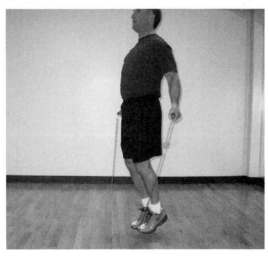

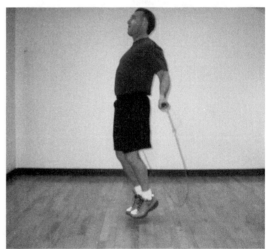

(b) 3 MINUTES OF AEROBIC EXERCISE

8. Abdominals/Legs: to be performed on a firm exercise mat.

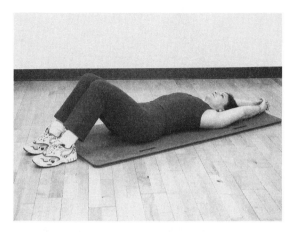

(a) SIT-UPS—30 to 40 reps

BEGINNER:
Lie on back with knees bent, feet flat on the floor with heels up against your mat, thumbs clasped, with arms fully extended behind your head. Slowly raise your body all the way up, bringing your chest toward your knees. Exhale while sitting up. Slowly lower body to starting position while inhaling and repeat.

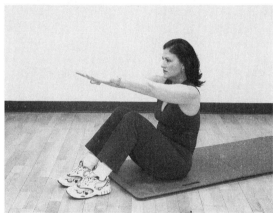

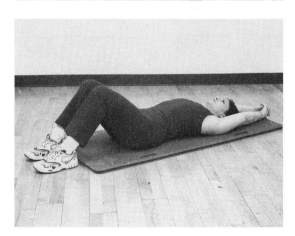

ADVANCED:

Lie on back with knees bent, feet flat on the floor with heels up against your mat, hands on your temples, palms facing in. Slowly raise your body all the way up, bringing your elbows toward your knees. Exhale while sitting up. Slowly lower body to starting position while inhaling and repeat.

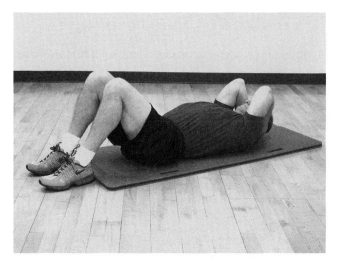

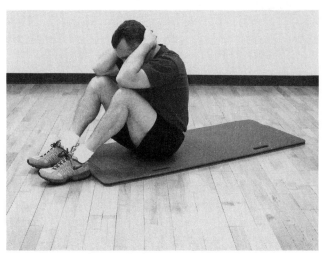

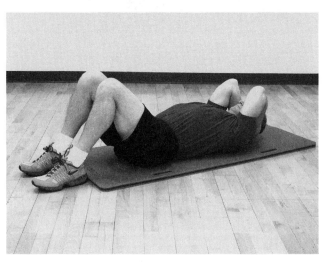

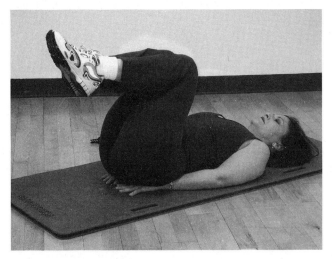

(b) LEG-OUTS—20 reps/20 reps

Lying on your back, with hands under buttocks, palms down, bring both knees in toward your chest. Slowly straighten legs out with toes pointed, and repeat. Inhale while bringing knees toward chest; exhale as you straighten legs. Beginners should straighten legs out at a higher angle. As you get stronger, try to bring legs lower to the ground (about two inches as illustrated) while straightening legs.

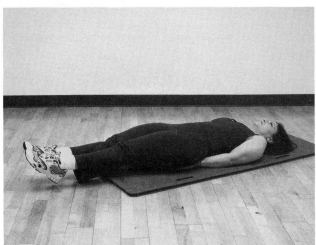

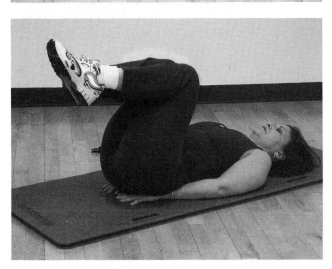

(c) ALTERNATES—20 reps/20 reps

Lie on your back with your hands under your buttocks or clasped behind your neck, with palms down, legs straight and toes pointed. Raise your right leg to a 90-degree angle, your left leg remaining near the floor. Pressing the small of your back into the floor, lower your right leg as you simultaneously lift your left leg to 90 degrees. Repeat this continuous scissoring motion.

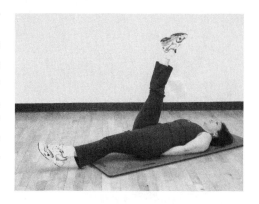

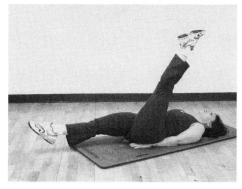

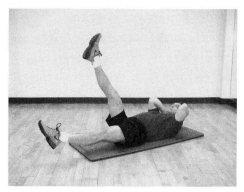

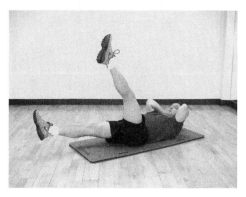

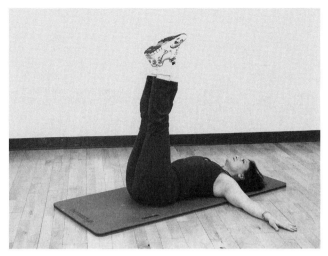

(d) V-SCISSORS (Women only)—20 reps/20 reps

Lie on your back, hands at your side or with hands under your buttocks with palms facing down. Raise both legs to 90 degrees. Pressing your back into the floor and with toes pointed and legs straight, slowly open legs as far as possible while exhaling. Bring legs back together, keeping toes pointed and legs straight as you inhale and repeat.

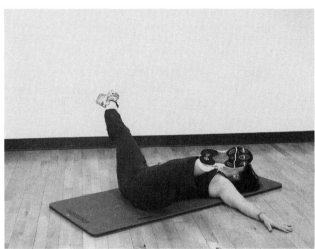

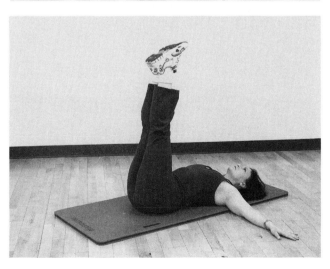

(e) KNEES TO CHEST—20 reps

Lie on back with arms extended, hands next to buttocks, palms down. Raise knees and feet in a tucked position toward chest, keeping lower back pressed against the floor while exhaling. Lower feet to ground while inhaling and repeat. Keep upper half of body motionless throughout movement.

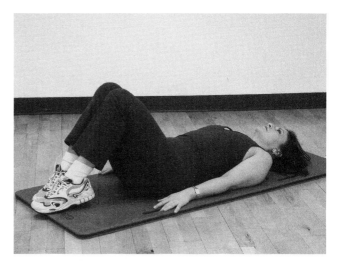

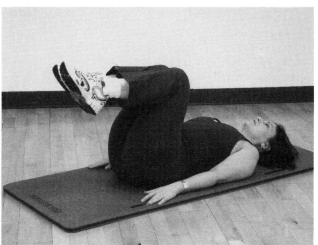

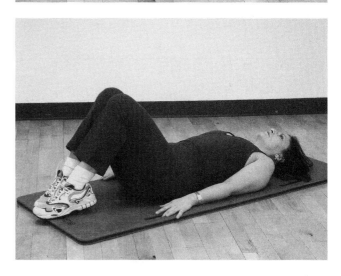

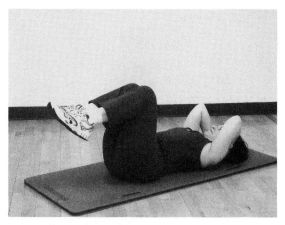

(f) ELBOWS TO KNEES—20 reps

Lying on back, raise knees and feet toward chest in a tucked position. Clasp your hands at the base of your neck. Gently curl your upper body, bringing your elbows toward knees, while exhaling. Slowly lower back and shoulders to mat while inhaling and repeat. Keep lower body motionless throughout entire movement.

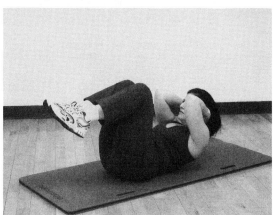

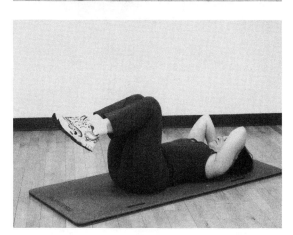

9. **Fat Burner**—**(a) jump rope or bounce on trampoline for 1 minute, then (b) 3 minutes of biking, walking jogging, or aerobic piece of your choice—with moderate intensity. (If unable to jump rope or use trampoline, do 4 minutes of aerobic of your choice.)**

(a) JUMPING ROPE—1 MINUTE

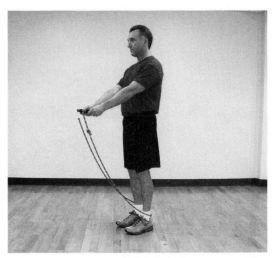

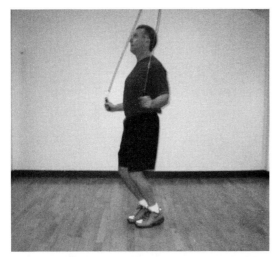

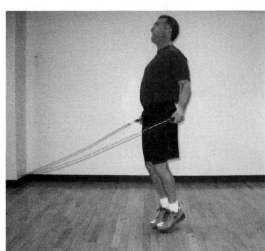

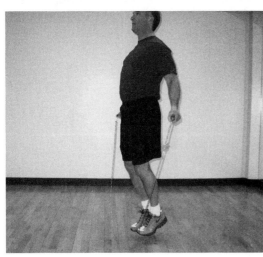

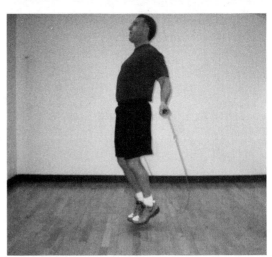

(b) 3 MINUTES OF AEROBIC EXERCISE

10. Jumping jacks—40 to 50 reps.

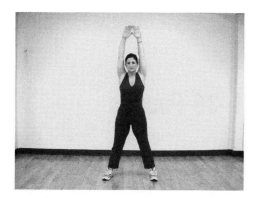

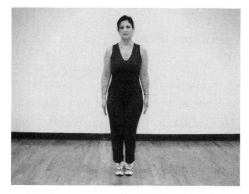

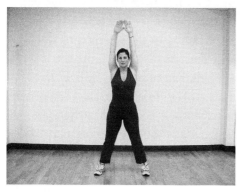

11. Cooldown—3 minutes of biking or walking leisurely.

Workout #2—See page 140 for Off Day Routine prescription.

CHAPTER SEVEN

Plans for Losing 11–30 Pounds

Most Important Factor in Diet Plans

This is often the easiest place to lose weight. The end is clearly in sight and the extra weight does not feel so overwhelming. It is important to stay focused and consistent. The two biggest mistakes people make here are getting too strict and getting too foolhardy. On the one hand, individuals in this category can often get so excited about reaching their goals that they will go a little overboard—exercising too much, eating too little—and before they know it, they have exhausted their bodies and their plan to speed up their weight loss has backfired—cravings come back stronger, they do not want to exercise, and they start overeating, and before they know it, the scale is heading in the wrong direction.

On the other hand, some individuals in this category get a little overexcited in a different way. They think *I'm not so far away from my goals; I can have an extra piece of pizza, an ice-cream cone, some chips,* et cetera. While eating these foods on rare occasions is acceptable, when you get careless it is easy to consume these "rewards" a little too often. Another thing to remember is that dessert is a "treat," not a treatment.

Helpful Tips for Successful Weight Reduction:

Keep a Food Journal—Write down what and when you eat and drink in a day and why: The journal will help you become aware of what you eat, will increase your control over eating, and will help you become aware of your eating patterns. Food becomes fattening when it is eaten for entertainment, comfort, or stress reduction.

Become Aware of Meal Timing: Eating earlier in the day prevents you from getting too hungry, losing control, and overeating in the evening.

Learn Your Calorie Budget: Know how much you can eat and still lose weight so you can be sure to fuel your body with an adequate amount of essential nutrients.

Eat Slowly: The brain needs about 20 minutes to receive the signal that you've eaten your fill. Practice by putting your fork down between bites and taking pauses throughout the meal.

Keep Away from Food Sources That Tempt You: Out of sight, out of mind, out of *mouth*! Hide high-calorie foods and keep healthy snacks readily available.

Taste Your Food: Calories should be tasted, not wasted. Do nothing else while eating and really savor your food.

*Please note: For those individuals who are vegetarian or have other special dietary needs, please log on to eatright.org or ediets.com to find a dietician near you.

Meal Plans for Losing 11–30 Pounds

Limited Approach
1400 CALORIES PER DAY
(221 GM CARBOHYDRATE, 80 GM PROTEIN, 44 GM FAT)

BREAKFAST *(400 calories, approx. 55 gm carbohydrate, 20 gm protein, 11 gm fat):*

1. **(400 calories, 57 gm carb, 14 gm protein, 10 gm fat)**

   1 1/2 cups whole grain cereal (unsweetened, ready-to-eat cereal)

   1 cup skim milk

   1 cup berries

   12 almonds

2. **(400 calories, 45 gm carb, 20 gm protein, 12 gm fat)**

   1/2 cup 1 percent cottage cheese

   1 cup berries

   12 almonds

   2 slices of whole grain bread

3. (400 calories, 55 gm carb, 18 gm protein, 8 gm fat)

   2 slices of whole grain bread

   1 tbs. peanut butter

   1 apple

   6 oz. low-fat yogurt

4. (400 calories, 53 gm carb, 20 gm protein, 10 gm fat)

   2 poached eggs

   2 slices of whole grain bread

   1 1/2 cups melon

5. (400 calories, 48 gm carb, 20 gm protein, 11 gm fat)

   1 cup cooked oatmeal

   9 chopped walnut halves

   1 chopped Red Delicious apple

   1/2 cup low-fat cottage cheese

6. (400 calories, 45 gm carb, 23 gm protein, 10 gm fat)

   Omelet—1 whole egg and 2 egg whites + 1/2 oz. low-fat cheese + 1/2 cup spinach

   2 slices of whole grain bread

   1 cup sliced strawberries

7. (400 calories, 50 gm carb, 19 gm protein, 11 gm fat)

   2 slices of whole grain bread

   1 1/2 oz. cheese

   1/2 cup sliced tomato

   1 cup mixed melon

LUNCH *(500 calories, approx. 68 gm carbohydrate, 25 gm protein, 14 gm fat):*

1. (500 calories, 65 gm carb, 22 gm protein, 15 gm fat)

   2 slices of whole grain bread

   2 oz. white meat turkey

   1/4 avocado

   1/2 cup sliced tomato and lettuce

   1/2 cup unsweetened applesauce with 1/4 cup low-fat granola

2. (500 calories, 65 gm carb, 22 gm protein, 15 gm fat)

   1 whole wheat pita

   2 oz. chunk white tuna fish

   3 tsps. mayonnaise

   1/2 cup mixed shredded carrots, lettuce, and celery

   24 cherries

3. (500 calories, 65 gm carb, 22 gm protein, 15 gm fat)

   2 oz. of cold chicken (cup up) mix with 3 tsps. mayonnaise

   2 slices of rye bread

   1/2 cup sliced tomato and lettuce

   1 whole diced mango

4. (500 calories, 65 gm carb, 25 gm protein, 15 gm fat)

   Big Salad:

   2 cups mixed greens

   1/2 cup diced carrots

   1/2 cup diced bell peppers

1/3 cup beans

2 oz. grilled chicken

4 chopped walnuts

1 diced apple

2 tbsps. vinaigrette salad dressing

1 medium nectarine

5. (500 calories, 70 gm carb, 24 gm protein, 15 gm fat)

2 oz. lean roast beef

2 slices of rye bread

1 tsp. mayonnaise

1/2 cup sliced tomato and lettuce

1/2 cup carrot sticks

1 1/2 cups fresh pineapple topped with 6 slivered almonds

6. (500 calories, 60 gm carb, 28 gm protein, 15 gm fat)

2 cups spinach

1 oz. feta cheese

1 oz. firm tofu

1/2 cup water chestnuts

1/2 cup snap peas

3/4 cup mandarin oranges

1 tbsp. reduced-fat ginger salad dressing

10 whole grain crackers

7. (500 calories, 65 gm carb, 28 gm protein, 15 gm fat)

2 slices of whole grain bread

2 oz. white meat turkey

1 oz. low-fat cheese

2 tsps. mayonnaise

1/2 cup sliced tomato and lettuce

1 1/2 cups mixed fruit salad

DINNER *(500 calories, approx. 68 gm carbohydrate, 25 gm protein, 14 gm fat):*

1. (500 calories, 65 gm carb, 26 gm protein, 15 gm fat)

2 oz. cooked chicken (no skin)

2/3 cup brown rice

1/2 cup green beans sautéed in 1 tsp. olive oil and 6 slivered almonds

1 cup mixed greens with 1/2 cup chopped tomatoes and 1/2 cup chopped peppers

1 tbsp. salad dressing

1 medium apple

2. (500 calories, 70 gm carb, 23 gm protein, 14 gm fat)

2 oz. lean cooked roast beef

1/3 cup brown rice

1/2 cup carrots

1/2 cup cauliflower

1 1/2 tsps. olive oil

1 whole grain dinner roll

1 orange

3. (500 calories, 68 gm carb, 29 gm protein, 14 gm fat)

2 oz. broiled salmon

1 large sweet potato

1 cup sautéed spinach with 1 1/2 tsps. olive oil

1 cup sliced tomato

$^1/_2$ cup diced melon

4. (500 calories, 50 gm carb, 25 gm protein, 14 gm fat)

   2 oz. sautéed shrimp in 1 $^1/_2$ tsps. olive oil

   1 cup whole wheat pasta

   $^1/_2$ cup jarred tomato sauce

   $^1/_2$ cup artichoke hearts

   1 $^1/_4$ cups sliced strawberries

5. (500 calories, 65 gm carb, 29 gm protein, 14 gm fat)

   3 oz. baked cod

   2 cups baked winter squash

   1 cup mixed greens (kale, collard, and mustard) sautéed in 2 $^1/_2$ tsps. olive oil

   2 cups cubed papaya

6. (500 calories, 70 gm carb, 27 gm protein, 14 gm fat)

   2 oz. flank steak

   1 cup whole wheat couscous

   2 cups roasted broccoli and cauliflower with 1 $^1/_2$ tsps. olive oil

   $^3/_4$ cup raspberries

7. (500 calories, 68 gm carb, 27 gm protein, 14 gm fat)

   2 oz. barbecued chicken

   1 medium corn on the cob

   $^2/_3$ cup baked beans

   1 $^1/_2$ cups cucumber and tomato salad tossed with 1 $^1/_2$ tbsps. olive oil–based dressing

   $^1/_2$ cup cubed watermelon

Dynamic Approach

1800 CALORIES PER DAY

(247 GM CARBOHYDRATE, 90 GM PROTEIN, 50 GM FAT)

BREAKFAST *(500 calories, approx. 68 gm carbohydrate, 25 gm protein, 14 gm fat):*

1. (500 calories, 72 gm carb, 24 gm protein, 15 gm fat)

   2 $^1/_4$ cups whole grain cereal (unsweetened, ready-to-eat cereal)

   1 cup skim milk

   1 cup berries

   12 almonds

   1 hard-boiled egg

2. (500 calories, 66 gm carb, 33 gm protein, 15 gm fat)

   $^1/_2$ cup 1 percent cottage cheese

   1 cup berries

   1 cup melon

   12 almonds

   2 tbsp. Grape-Nuts

   1 slice of whole grain bread

   1 tsp. peanut butter

3. (500 calories, 67 gm carb, 26 gm protein, 13 gm fat)

   2 slices of whole grain bread

   1 tbs. peanut butter

1 apple

12 oz. low-fat yogurt

4. (500 calories, 65 gm carb, 28 gm protein, 15 gm fat)

2 poached eggs

2 slices of whole grain bread

3/4 cup plain low-fat yogurt

1 1/2 cups melon

5. (500 calories, 63 gm carb, 23 gm protein, 15 gm fat)

1 1/2 cups cooked oatmeal

12 chopped walnut halves

1 chopped Red Delicious apple

1/2 cup low-fat cottage cheese

6. (500 calories, 65 gm carb, 25 gm protein, 10 gm fat)

Omelet—1 whole egg and 2 egg whites + 1/2 oz. of low-fat cheese + 1/2 cup spinach + 1/2 cup chopped tomato

2 slices of whole grain bread

1 cup sliced strawberries

1 sliced kiwi

7. (500 calories, 65 gm carb, 22 gm protein, 16 gm fat)

2 slices of whole grain bread

2 oz. cheese

1/2 cup sliced tomato

2 cups mixed melon

LUNCH *(500 calories, approx. 68 gm carbohydrate, 25 gm protein, 14 gm fat):*

1. (500 calories, 65 gm carb, 22 gm protein, 15 gm fat)

2 slices of whole grain bread

2 oz. white meat turkey

1/4 avocado

1/2 cup sliced tomato and lettuce

1/2 cup unsweetened apple sauce with 1/4 cup low-fat granola

2. (500 calories, 65 gm carb, 22 gm protein, 15 gm fat)

1 whole wheat pita

2 oz. chunk white tuna fish

3 tsps. mayonnaise

1/2 cup mixed shredded carrots, lettuce, and celery

24 cherries

3. (500 calories, 65 gm carb, 22 gm protein, 15 gm fat)

2 oz. of cold chicken (cut up) mixed with 3 tsps. mayonnaise

2 slices of rye bread

1/2 cup sliced tomato and lettuce

1 whole diced mango

4. (500 calories, 65 gm carb, 25 gm protein, 15 gm fat)

Big Salad:

2 cups mixed greens

1/2 cup diced carrots

1/2 cup diced bell peppers

1/3 cup beans

2 oz. grilled chicken

4 chopped walnuts

1 diced apple

2 tbsps. vinaigrette salad dressing

1 medium nectarine

5. (500 calories, 70 gm carb, 24 gm protein, 15 gm fat)

2 oz. lean roast beef

2 slices of rye bread

1 tsp. mayonnaise

1/2 cup sliced tomato and lettuce

1/2 cup carrot sticks

1 1/2 cups fresh pineapple topped with 6 slivered almonds

6. (500 calories, 60 gm carb, 28 gm protein, 15 gm fat)

2 cups spinach

1 oz. feta cheese

1 oz. firm tofu

1/2 cup water chestnuts

1/2 cup snap peas

3/4 cup mandarin oranges

1 tbsp. reduced-fat ginger salad dressing

10 whole grain crackers

7. (500 calories, 65 gm carb, 28 gm protein, 15 gm fat)

2 slices of whole grain bread

2 oz. white meat turkey

1 oz. low-fat cheese

2 tsps. mayonnaise

1/2 cup sliced tomato and lettuce

1 1/2 cups mixed fruit salad

SNACK (200 calories, approx. 27 gm carbohydrate, 10 gm protein, 6 gm fat):

1. (200 calories, 27 gm carb, 8 gm protein, 5 gm fat)

1 cup plain nonfat yogurt

3/4 cup fresh blackberries

6 chopped almonds

2. (200 calories, 27 gm carb, 8 gm protein, 5 gm fat)

1 medium apple

2 tsps. peanut butter

1 cup skim milk

3. (200 calories, 30 gm carb, 7 gm protein, 7 gm fat)

1 whole grain English muffin

1 oz. Swiss cheese

4. (200 calories, 27 gm carb, 8 gm protein, 5 gm fat)

Peanut-butter-and-jelly smoothie: Blend 1 cup skim milk + 1 1/4 cups fresh or frozen strawberries + 2 tsps. peanut butter

5. (200 calories, 27 gm carb, 8 gm protein, 5 gm fat)

six-inch whole wheat pita

1 sliced apple

2 tsps. peanut butter

6. (200 calories, 27 gm carb, 8 gm protein, 5 gm fat)

1 slice whole wheat raisin bread topped with 1 sliced kiwi and 1/4 cup ricotta cheese

7. (200 calories, 27 gm carb, 8 gm protein,
   5 gm fat)

   1/2 six-inch whole wheat pita

   1/3 cup hummus

   1/2 cup carrot sticks

DINNER *(600 calories, approx. 85 gm carbohydrate, 30 gm protein, 16 gm fat):*

1. (600 calories, 85 gm carb, 28 gm protein,
   15 gm fat)

   2 oz. cooked chicken (no skin)

   1 cup brown rice

   1 cup green beans sautéed in 1 tsp. olive oil
       and 6 slivered almonds

   1 cup mixed greens with 1/2 cup chopped
       tomatoes and 1/2 cup chopped
       peppers

   1 tbsp. salad dressing

   1 medium apple

2. (600 calories, 85 gm carb, 26 gm protein,
   16 gm fat)

   2 oz. lean cooked roast beef

   2/3 cup brown rice

   1/2 cup carrots

   1/2 cup cauliflower

   2 tsps. olive oil

   1 whole grain dinner roll

   1 orange

3. (600 calories, 83 gm carb, 29 gm protein,
   16 gm fat)

   2 oz. broiled salmon

   1 large sweet potato

   1 cup sautéed spinach with 2 tsps. olive oil

   1 cup sliced tomato

   1 1/2 cups diced melon

4. (600 calories, 85 gm carb, 30 gm protein, 16
   gm fat)

   2 oz. sautéed shrimp in 2 tsps. olive oil

   1 1/2 cups whole wheat pasta

   1/2 cup jarred tomato sauce

   1/2 cup artichoke hearts

   1/2 cup spinach

   1 1/4 cups sliced strawberries

   1 sliced fresh peach

5. (600 calories, 85 gm carb, 32 gm protein,
   16 gm fat)

   3 oz. baked cod

   1/3 cup cooked whole wheat couscous

   2 cups baked winter squash

   1 cup mixed greens (kale, collard, and mus-
       tard) sautéed in 3 tsps. olive oil

   2 cups cubed papaya

6. (600 calories, 85 gm carb, 27 gm protein,
   16 gm fat)

   2 oz. flank steak

   1 cup whole wheat couscous

   2 cups roasted broccoli and cauliflower with
       2 tsps. olive oil

   1 1/2 cups raspberries

7. (500 calories, 83 gm carb, 27 gm protein, 16 gm fat)

   2 oz. barbecued chicken

   1 medium corn on the cob

1 cup baked beans

1 1/2 cups cucumber and tomato salad tossed with 2 tbsps. olive oil–based dressing

1/2 cup cubed watermelon

Balanced Approach
1600 CALORIES PER DAY
(221 GM CARBOHYDRATE, 80 GM PROTEIN, 44 GM FAT)

BREAKFAST (400 calories, approx. 55 gm carbohydrate, 20 gm protein, 11 gm fat):

1. (400 calories, 57 gm carb, 14 gm protein, 10 gm fat)

   1 1/2 cups whole grain cereal (unsweetened, ready-to-eat cereal)

   1 cup skim milk

   1 cup berries

   12 almonds

2. (400 calories, 45 gm carb, 20 gm protein, 12 gm fat)

   1/2 cup 1 percent cottage cheese

   1 cup berries

   12 almonds

   2 slices of whole grain bread

3. (400 calories, 55 gm carb, 18 gm protein, 8 gm fat)

   2 slices of whole grain bread

   1 tbsp. peanut butter

   1 apple

   6 oz. low-fat yogurt

4. (400 calories, 53 gm carb, 20 gm protein, 10 gm fat)

   2 poached eggs

2 slices of whole grain bread

1 1/2 cups melon

5. (400 calories, 48 gm carb, 20 gm protein, 11 gm fat)

   1 cup cooked oatmeal

   9 chopped walnut halves

   1 chopped Red Delicious apple

   1/2 cup low-fat cottage cheese

6. (400 calories, 45 gm carb, 23 gm protein, 10 gm fat)

   Omelet—1 whole egg and 2 egg whites + 1/2 oz. of low-fat cheese + 1/2 cup spinach

   2 slices of whole grain bread

   1 cup sliced strawberries

7. (400 calories, 50 gm carb, 19 gm protein, 10 gm fat)

   2 slices of whole grain bread

   1 1/2 oz. cheese

   1/2 cup sliced tomato

   1 cup mixed melon

LUNCH *(500 calories, approx. 68 gm carbohydrate, 25 gm protein, 14 gm fat):*

1. **(500 calories, 65 gm carb, 22 gm protein, 15 gm fat)**

   2 slices of whole grain bread

   2 oz. white meat turkey

   1/4 avocado

   1/2 cup sliced tomato and lettuce

   1/2 cup unsweetened apple sauce with
       1/4 cup low-fat granola

2. **(500 calories, 65 gm carb, 22 gm protein, 15 gm fat)**

   1 whole wheat pita

   2 oz. chunk white tuna fish

   3 tsps. mayonnaise

   1/2 cup mixed shredded carrots, lettuce, and
       celery

   24 cherries

3. **(500 calories, 65 gm carb, 22 gm protein, 15 gm fat)**

   2 oz. of cold chicken (cut up) mixed with
       3 tsps. mayonnaise

   2 slices of rye bread

   1/2 cup sliced tomato and lettuce

   1 whole diced mango

4. **(500 calories, 65 gm carb, 25 gm protein, 15 gm fat)**

   Big Salad:

       2 cups mixed greens

       1/2 cup diced carrots

       1/2 cup diced bell peppers

       1/3 cup beans

       2 oz. grilled chicken

       4 chopped walnuts

       1 diced apple

       2 tbsps. vinaigrette salad dressing

   1 medium nectarine

5. **(500 calories, 70 gm carb, 24 gm protein, 15 gm fat)**

   2 oz. lean roast beef

   2 slices of rye bread

   1 tsp. mayonnaise

   1/2 cup sliced tomato and lettuce

   1/2 cup carrot sticks

   1 1/2 cups fresh pineapple topped with
       6 slivered almonds

6. **(500 calories, 60 gm carb, 28 gm protein, 15 gm fat)**

   2 cups spinach

   1 oz. feta cheese

   1 oz. firm tofu

   1/2 cup water chestnuts

   1/2 cup snap peas

   3/4 cup mandarin oranges

   1 tbsp. reduced-fat ginger salad dressing

   10 whole grain crackers

7. **(500 calories, 65 gm carb, 28 gm protein, 15 gm fat)**

   2 slices of whole grain bread

   2 oz. white meat turkey

   1 oz. low-fat cheese

   2 tsps. mayonnaise

   1/2 cup sliced tomato and lettuce

   1 1/2 cups mixed fruit salad

SNACK *(200 calories, approx. 27 gm carbohydrate, 10 gm protein, 6 gm fat):*

1. (200 calories, 27 gm carb, 8 gm protein, 5 gm fat)

   1 cup plain nonfat yogurt

   3/4 cup fresh blackberries

   6 chopped almonds

2. (200 calories, 27 gm carb, 8 gm protein, 5 gm fat)

   1 medium apple

   2 tsps. peanut butter

   1 cup skim milk

3. (200 calories, 30 gm carb, 7 gm protein, 7 gm fat)

   1 whole grain English muffin

   1 oz. Swiss cheese

4. (200 calories, 27 gm carb, 8 gm protein, 5 gm fat)

   Peanut-butter-and-jelly smoothie: Blend 1 cup skim milk + 1 1/4 cups fresh or frozen strawberries + 2 tsps. peanut butter

5. (200 calories, 27 gm carb, 8 gm protein, 5 gm fat)

   six-inch whole wheat pita

   1 sliced apple

   2 tsps. peanut butter

6. (200 calories, 27 gm carb, 8 gm protein, 5 gm fat)

   1 slice whole wheat raisin bread topped with 1 sliced kiwi and 1/4 cup ricotta cheese

7. (200 calories, 27 gm carb, 8 gm protein, 5 gm fat)

   1/2 six-inch whole wheat pita

   1/3 cup hummus

   1/2 cup carrot sticks

DINNER *(500 calories, approx. 68 gm carbohydrate, 25 gm protein, 14 gm fat):*

1. (500 calories, 65 gm carb, 26 gm protein, 15 gm fat)

   2 oz. cooked chicken (no skin)

   2/3 cup brown rice

   1/2 cup green beans sautéed in 1 tsp. olive oil and 6 slivered almonds

   1 cup mixed greens with 1/2 cup chopped tomatoes and 1/2 cup chopped peppers

   1 tbsp. salad dressing

   1 medium apple

2. (500 calories, 70 gm carb, 23 gm protein, 14 gm fat)

   2 oz. lean cooked roast beef

   1/3 cup brown rice

   1/2 cup carrots

   1/2 cup cauliflower

   1 1/2 tsps. olive oil

   1 whole grain dinner roll

   1 orange

3. (500 calories, 68 gm carb, 29 gm protein, 14 gm fat)

   2 oz. broiled salmon

   1 large sweet potato

   1 cup sautéed spinach with 1 $^1/_2$ tsps. olive oil

   1 cup sliced tomato

   $^1/_2$ cup diced melon

4. (500 calories, 50 gm carb, 25 gm protein, 14 gm fat)

   2 oz. sautéed shrimp with 1 $^1/_2$ tsps. olive oil

   1 cup whole-wheat pasta

   $^1/_2$ cup jarred tomato sauce

   $^1/_2$ cup artichoke hearts

   1 $^1/_4$ cups sliced strawberries

5. (500 calories, 65 gm carb, 29 gm protein, 14 gm fat)

   3 oz. baked cod

   2 cups baked winter squash

   1 cup mixed greens (kale, collard, and mustard) sautéed in 2 $^1/_2$ tsps. olive oil

   2 cups cubed papaya

6. (500 calories, 70 gm carb, 27 gm protein, 14 gm fat)

   2 oz. flank steak

   1 cup whole wheat couscous

   2 cups roasted broccoli and cauliflower with 1 $^1/_2$ tsps. olive oil

   $^3/_4$ cup raspberries

7. (500 calories, 68 gm carb, 27 gm protein, 14 gm fat)

   2 oz. barbecued chicken

   1 medium corn on the cob

   $^2/_3$ cup baked beans

   1 $^1/_2$ cups cucumber and tomato salad tossed with 1 $^1/_2$ tbsps. olive oil based dressing

   $^1/_2$ cup cubed watermelon

Additional Foods to Choose as Between Meal Snacks

LOW-CALORIE

Fresh fruit

Fresh vegetables (can dip them in 2 tbsps. hummus, salsa, or homemade low-fat dip)

Low-fat yogurt

Low-fat cottage cheese

Hot-air-popped popcorn

$^1/_4$ cup dry-roasted nuts (need to limit portions)

2 tsps. peanut butter + 2 graham crackers + 2 tsp. jam

1 oz. of reduced-fat cheese with 10 whole grain crackers

1 slice of reduced-fat cheese melted over tomato on whole grain bread

Non-fat Greek yogurt with 1 cup of berries and 2 tbsps. chopped nuts

$^1/_4$ cup dry-roasted mixed nuts (almonds, pumpkinseeds, walnuts)

MEDIUM-CALORIE

1 tbsp. nut butter on a slice of whole wheat bread

1 tbsp. nut butter on a medium apple

$^{1}/_{2}$ whole wheat English muffin + 1 slice low-fat mozzarella cheese + 1 tbsp. marinara sauce

1 medium orange diced into 1 serving of oatmeal + 2 walnut halves

FOR SWEET CRAVINGS
Fresh watermelon

Fresh berries

Sugar-free Jell-O

Fat-free/sugar-free fudge pop

Sugar-free Popsicle

FOR SAVORY CRAVINGS
Fresh-vegetables dipped in salsa

Hot-air popped popcorn

Exercise Prescription for Losing 11–30 Pounds

Most Important Factor
As you get nearer your goal of your "ideal weight," your caloric intake becomes just as important as your exercise frequency. But the most important factor for you to focus on with regard to your exercise regimen, aside from being consistent, is the *intensity* at which you work out. For each hour you devote to working out, the more intensely you exercise, the more calories you will burn in the same amount of time. As you become more fit, you must also be conscious of your total caloric intake, ensuring that you are creating a deficit of calories that will enable you to maintain weight loss.

Fitness Equipment Needed
1. **Choose one:** recumbent or upright stationary bike, treadmill, elliptical machine, cross trainer, or, if no access to a piece of aerobic equipment, walk/jog instead

2. Firm exercise mat

3. A lightweight (2–4 lb.) collapsible aerobic toning bar for both men and women

4. A 10–15 lb. weighted bar for men

5. A lightweight speed or beaded jump rope

   (See page 179 for photos of fitness equipment needed.)

While jumping rope, make sure you are doing so on a surface that has a give to it such as a wooden floor, short grass, a rubberized track or tennis court, or the like. *Do not* jump rope on asphalt or cement. If you don't have access to this type of surface and/or need help in improving your jump rope skills, log onto *www.exude.com* to view Jump Rope Mat and Jumping Rope Videos.

Please Note: All of the following exercise regimens can be performed at home, at your gym, or even while traveling.

Exercise Regimen
Frequency—2, 3, 4, or 5 days per week
Duration—60 minutes
****Before starting this or any exercise program, get your doctor's approval.*

Workout #1
Full-Body Routine—2–3 days per week, every other day, Mondays, Wednesdays, and Fridays or Tuesday, Thursdays, and Saturdays.

"Reps" = Repetitions; the number of times you actually perform the exercise.

1. **Warm-up**—bike, brisk walk, elliptical machine, or cross trainer for 25 minutes, with low to moderate resistance, 90 + RPMs, or walk at 4.0 MPH or jog at 5.5 + MPH with no incline.

2. **Stretch**—3 minutes.

3. **Fat Burner**—(a) squat thrusts: 10 to 20 reps, then perform side benders for 50 to 60 reps to catch breath; (b) jump rope or bike or perform any other aerobic activity of your choice for 3 minutes.

4. **Upper Body Exercises**—with aerobic toning bar for women, 10-15 lb. weighted bar for men; (a) push-outs: 40 to 50 reps; (b) behind the neck press: 40 to 50 reps; (c) front press: 40 to 50 reps; (d) upright rows: 40 to 50 reps; (e) curls: 40 to 50 reps; (f) kick-backs: 30 reps, rest 30 seconds, repeat 20 reps.

5. **Jumping Jacks**—60 to 75 reps.

6. **Fat Burner**—(a) squat thrusts: 10 to 20 reps, then perform side benders for 50 to 60 reps to catch breath; (b) jump rope or bike or perform any other aerobic activity of your choice for 3 minutes.

7. **Legs/Hips**—(a) standing knee to opposite chest: 40 reps; (b) L kicks: 40 reps; (c) march in place on toes: 75 reps.

8. **Abdominals/Legs**—(a) sit-ups: 50 reps; (b) leg-outs: 40 to 50 reps; (c) V-scissors: 40 reps; (d) alternates: 60 reps; (e) elbows to knees: 35 reps; (f) knees to elbows: 35 reps; (g) repeat sit-ups: 25 reps.

9. **Fat Burner**—jump rope for 5–10 minutes or bike or perform any other aerobic activity of your choice for 10 minutes—vigorously!

10. **Cooldown**—easy biking or walking for 3 minutes.

If you need a break at any time during your exercise regimen, you can simply get on a stationary bike or any other piece of aerobic equipment or walk for 1–3 minutes to allow your heart rate to come down safely *before* you resume. Also, if you want to pay more attention to either your upper body, midsection, or lower body, you can perform either more repetitions or do an extra set of exercises that target that region.

Based upon your time allotment and level of fitness, you can either cool down or perform another upper body routine, #4, and/or another set of abdominals/legs, #8, and then cool down. For every exercise, try to add 1–2 repetitions each two weeks and build up to 75 reps for all exercises. Aerobically, try to increase your jumping rope to 15 minutes of continuous jumping without taking a break. If you cannot jump rope due to a medical or orthopedic concern, increase your speed and resistance slightly to ensure that you're working intensely enough during all aerobic exercises.

Workout #2 (Optional, depending upon which approach you choose: Balanced or Dynamic)

Off Day Routine—2 to 3 days per week on days in between Full-Body Routines.

1. Aerobic exercise of your choice for 40 minutes.

2. Stretch—3 minutes.

3. Legs/hips—(a) standing knee to opposite chest: 40 reps; (b) L kicks: 40 reps; (e) march in place on toes: 75 reps.

4. Abdominals/legs—(a) sit-ups: 60 reps; (b) leg-outs: 40 reps; (c) V scissors: 35; (d) alternates: 60; (e) elbows to knees: 35; (f) knees to elbows: 35 reps.

5. Cooldown—nice and easy for 3 minutes of biking, walking, or the like.

---

3. Collapsible Aerobic Toning Bar

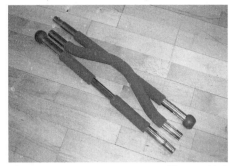

Unassembled

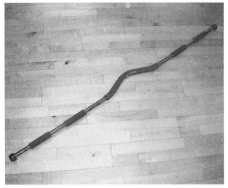

Assembled

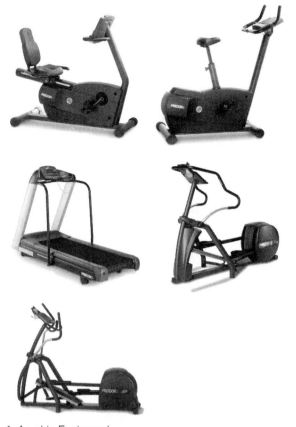

1. Aerobic Equipment

4. Weighted Bar

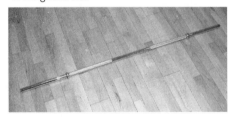

2. Firm Exercise Mat

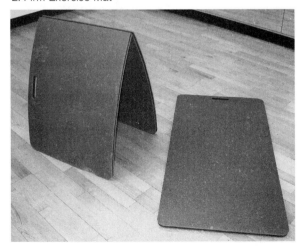

5. Speed and Beaded Jump Rope.

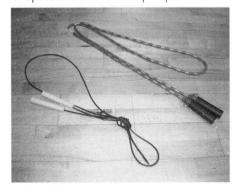

Workout #1—Full-Body Routine

1. Warm-up—25 minutes

2. Stretch: hold each stretch for 30–60 seconds.

ARM CIRCLES

With arms outstretched, slowly circle your arms backward for 5 revolutions and then forward for 5 revolutions.

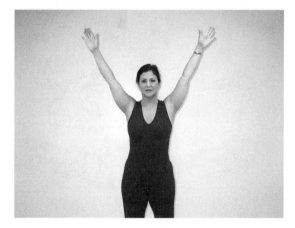

TRICEPS

With arms overhead, gently pull the left elbow behind your head with your right hand. Hold when you reach a comfortable stretch in the rear shoulder and upper back. Switch arms and repeat.

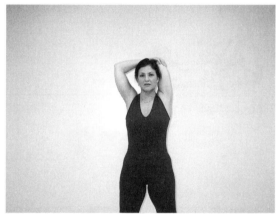

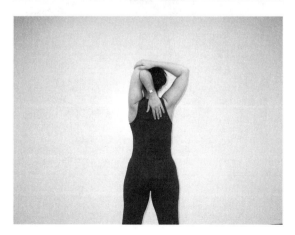

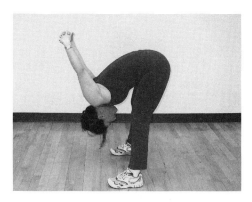

SHOULDERS, CHEST, AND HAMSTRINGS

Grasp hands behind your back, with palms facing each other. Slightly bend your knees and lift arms up as you bend forward at the waist. Hold when you feel a comfortable stretch in the shoulders, chest, and hamstrings.

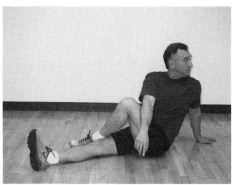

SPINAL TWIST

Keeping the right leg straight, left arm behind for support, cross left leg over and place foot outside the right knee. With the right hand or elbow on the left knee, slowly twist and look over your left shoulder while simultaneously pulling the knee in the opposite direction; hold. You will feel pressure in the hip, side, and upper back. Repeat on opposite side.

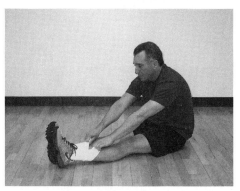

HAMSTRINGS

With legs straight, ankles flexed, bend forward from the hips and reach out toward your toes and, based on your flexibility, grab on to either your socks or shoelaces while holding the stretch. You will feel tension just behind the knees, in the upper calves, and in the lower back area. If possible, you should also perform this stretch with legs apart, using the preceding instructions.

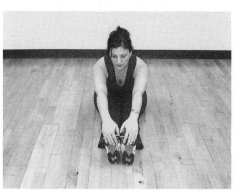

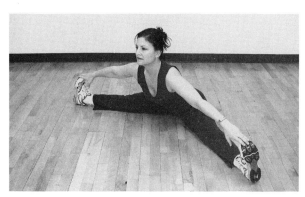

GROIN

In sitting position, pull your soles of your feet together and grab hold of your ankles. Gently pull heels toward the groin area. Let your knees relax toward the floor and gently press your elbows down on your knees to increase the stretch.

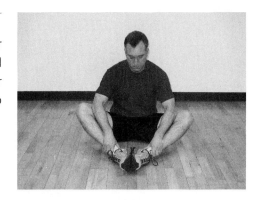

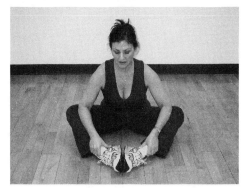

QUADRICEPS

Lie down on your left side. Bend your right leg and grab your right ankle with your right hand. Gently pull your right leg back toward your buttocks. Hold the position when you feel a comfortable stretch in front of your right thigh. Release slowly and roll over to your left side and repeat.

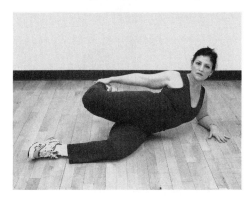

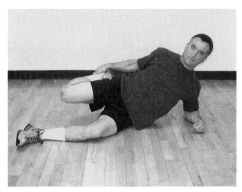

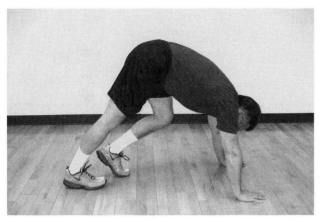

CALVES #1

With hands and knees on all fours, straighten your body into a **V** position. With both feet together, bend your left knee and press your right heel toward the ground, stretching your right calf. Repeat on other side.

OR

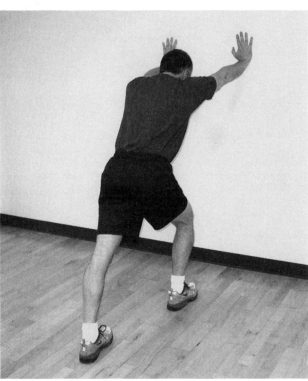

CALVES #2

Stand a little farther than arm's length away from a wall or solid support, lean on it with hands placed shoulder distance away. Bring one foot forward, knee bent, while keeping the back leg straight, heel pressing into the floor. Lean toward wall while holding stretch. Switch legs and repeat.

3. **Fat Burner–(a)** squat thrusts: 10 to 20 reps, then perform side benders for 50 to 60 reps to catch breath; **(b)** jump rope for 3 minutes or bike or perform any other aerobic activity of your choice, vigorously!

(a) SQUAT THRUSTS—10 to 20 reps

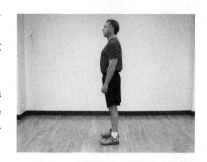

i. Stand with back straight, knees slightly flexed, and feet shoulder width apart.

ii. Bending knees approximately seventy-five degrees into a squat position (keep thighs parallel with the floor), place palms facedown 8 inches in front of toes and slightly wider than shoulder width.

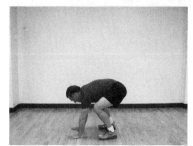

iii. Exhaling, kick both legs out behind you, landing toes on the floor and legs fully straight and extended.

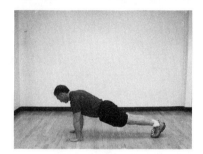

iv. Thrust back to position ii, then stand up with back straight as you inhale to position i.

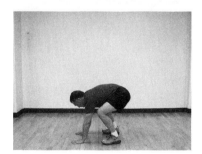

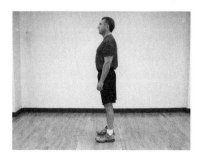

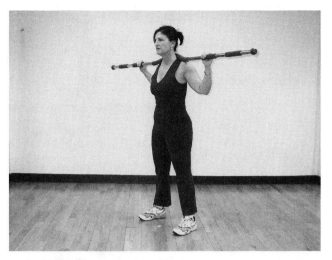

SIDE BENDERS—50 to 60 reps

Rest after squat thrusts by doing side benders until you catch your breath.

i. Rest the aerobic toning bar across your shoulders and slowly bend your upper body from side to side.

ii. Keep your lower body still, moving only at the waist.

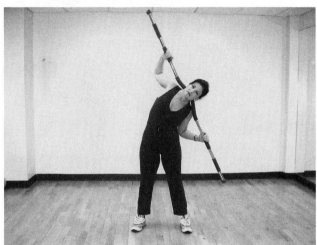

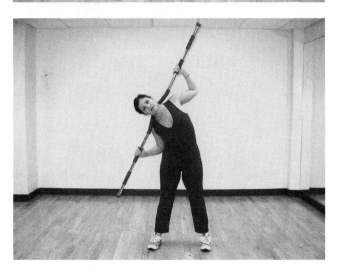

(b) JUMPING ROPE—3 MINUTES

How to Jump Rope:

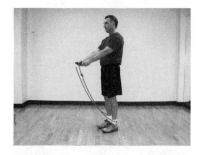

i. Practice swinging rope overhead without jumping, forming a loop.

ii. Move forearms in time with feet.

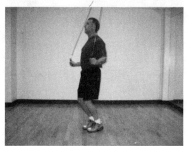

iii. Jump just high enough for rope to pass under feet (one inch off the ground). Jump with both feet at once. (Jumping higher than one inch will create unnecessary stress on the legs, increasing the potential for injury.)

iv. Rope should hit the round about one foot in front of feet with each revolution.

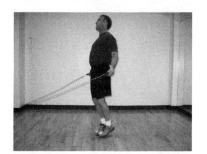

v. Caution: Avoid double jumping. Your workout will not be as effective! After each jump the rope should pass under your feet.

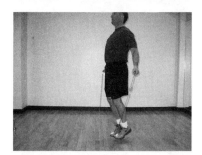

OR 3 MINUTES OF AEROBIC EXERCISE

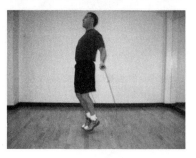

4. Upper Body Exercises—with aerobic toning bar for women and a weighted bar for men.

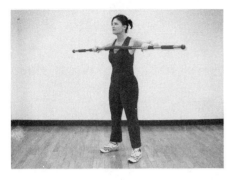

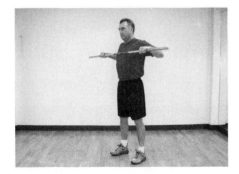

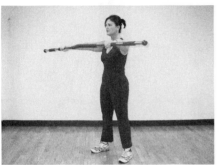

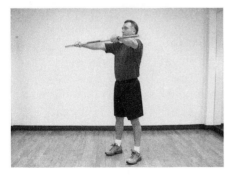

(a) PUSH-OUTS—40 to 50 reps

6

Keep back straight, knees slightly flexed, and feet shoulder width apart.

i. Grip bar, palms facing down, just past shoulder width. Raise bar up just above your chest line with elbows up and wrists firm.

ii. Extend arms straight out, holding bar above chest level, and exhale.

iii. While inhaling, bring bar back to starting position and repeat. Keep lower body aligned and still throughout entire exercise.

iv. Moderate speed throughout entire movement.

(b) BEHIND THE NECK PRESS—40 to 50 reps

Keep back straight, knees slightly flexed, and feet shoulder width apart.

i. Grip bar just past shoulder width and place behind neck and shoulders.

ii. Fully extend arms and raise bar straight up behind head while exhaling. Bend arms and slowly return bar to behind neck while inhaling and repeat.

iii. Slow speed throughout entire movement.

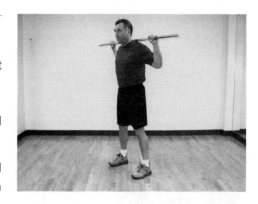

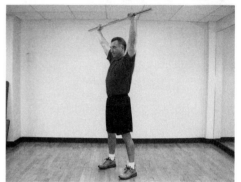

(c) FRONT PRESS—40 to 50 reps

Keep back straight, knees slightly flexed, and feet shoulder width apart.

i. Grip bar just past shoulder width and rest bar across top of chest.

ii. Fully extend arms upwards and raise bar straight up while exhaling. Bend arms and slowly return bar to top of chest while inhaling and repeat.

iii. Moderate speed throughout entire movement.

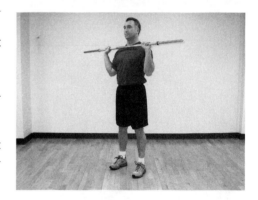

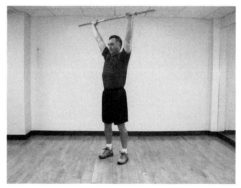

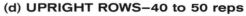

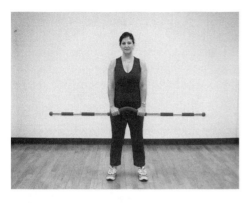

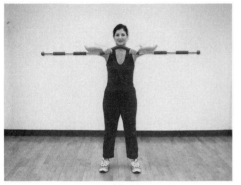

(d) UPRIGHT ROWS—40 to 50 reps

Keep back straight, knees slightly flexed, and feet shoulder width apart.

i. Grip bar, palms facing down, six to eight inches apart. Hold bar with arms fully extended at front of thighs.

ii. Slowly raise bar to chin, keeping elbows at or above bar level while exhaling. Return to starting position while inhaling and repeat.

iii. Moderate speed throughout entire movement.

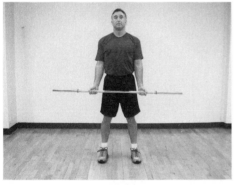

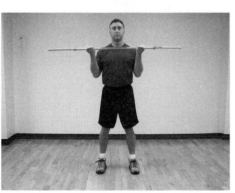

(e) CURLS—40 to 50 reps

Keep back straight, knees slightly flexed, and feet shoulder width apart.

i. Grip bar, palms facing up and shoulder width apart. Hold bar with arms fully extended at front of thighs.

ii. Keeping elbows stationary and wrists firm, curl bar up to chest while exhaling. Slowly extend arms and return bar to start position while inhaling and repeat.

iii. Moderate speed throughout entire movement.

(f) KICK-BACKS—30 reps/20 reps

Keep back straight, knees slightly flexed and feet shoulder width apart.

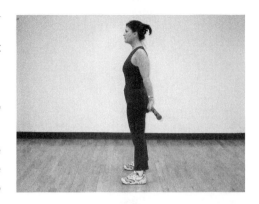

i.   Grip bar with arms fully extended at buttocks, palms facing outward about shoulder width apart.

ii. Keeping elbows stationary and wrists firm, raise bar away from your buttocks as far as possible while exhaling. Keeping arms straight, lower bar to buttocks while inhaling and repeat.

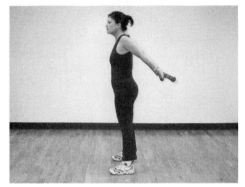

iii. Moderate speed throughout entire movement.

5. Jumping Jacks—60 to 75 reps.

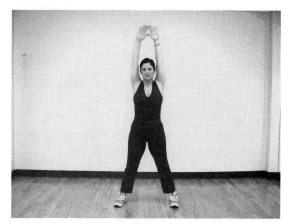

Start with arms extended fully overhead and legs apart. While exhaling, simultaneously bring arms down and touch hands on each side of the outside of thighs while shuffling feet together, barely lifting feet off the ground. Inhale as you return to starting position and repeat, keeping arms as straight as possible during entire movement.

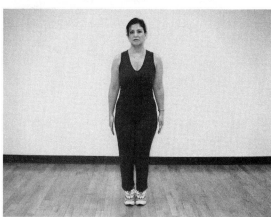

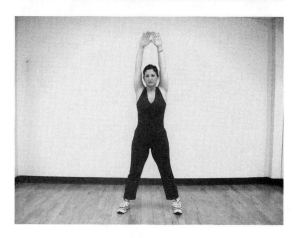

6. Fat Burner—(a) squat thrusts: 10 to 20 reps, then perform 50 to 60 side benders to catch breath; **(b)** jump rope for 3 minutes or bike or perform any other aerobic activity of your choice, vigorously!

(a) SQUAT THRUSTS–10 to 20 reps

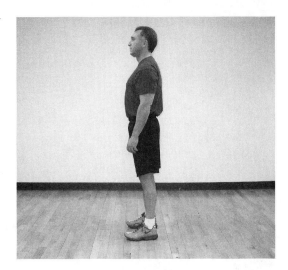

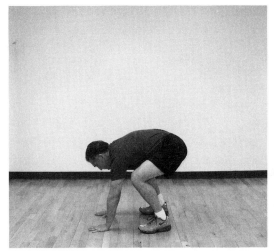

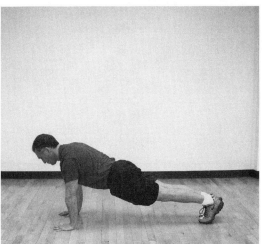

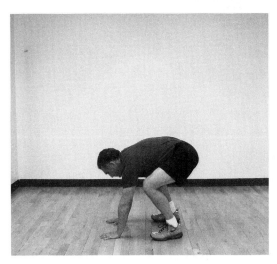

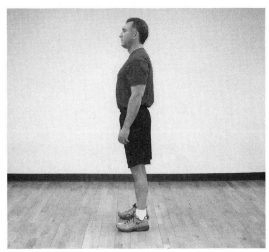

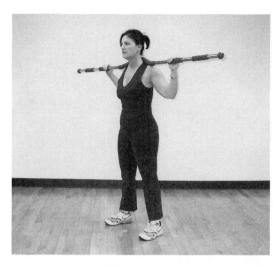

SIDE BENDERS–50 to 60 reps

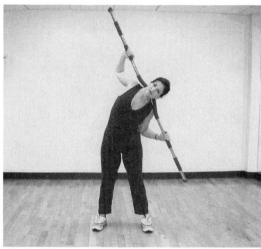

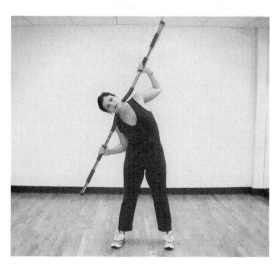

(b) JUMP ROPE–3 MINUTES

OR 3 MINUTES OF AEROBIC EXERCISE

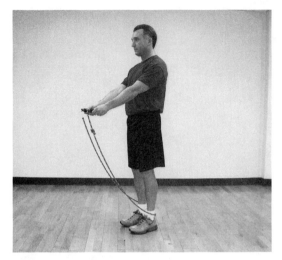

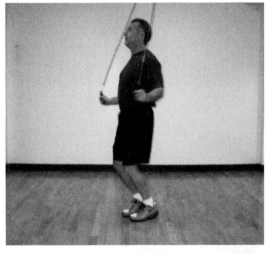

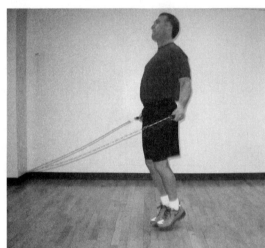

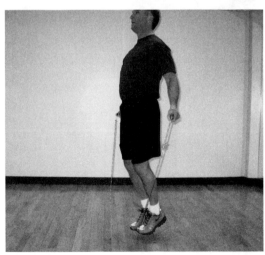

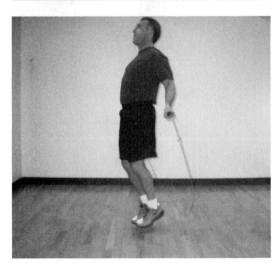

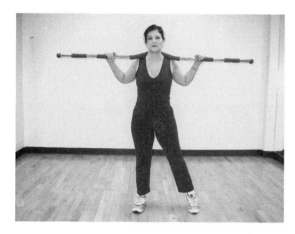

(a) STANDING KNEE TO OPPOSITE CHEST—40 reps

Rest the aerobic toning bar on your neck across your shoulders, with feet shoulder width apart.

i.   Transfer all weight to your right leg.
ii. Raise left knee up toward your right chest to at least waist level.
iii. Lower left foot to starting position, touching the ground, while keeping your weight on your right leg throughout the movement. Switch legs and repeat.
iv. Try to keep aerobic bar straight across back/shoulders while performing exercise.

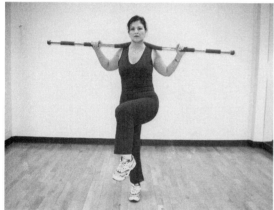

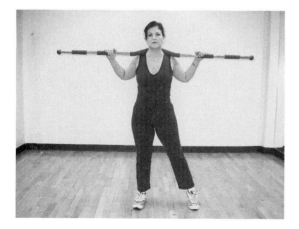

(b) L KICKS—40 reps

Hold the aerobic toning bar upright with your right hand and place your left hand on your waist.

i.   Start by raising your left leg and trying to get it to waist level, keeping it as straight as possible, pointing your toe without leaning your weight on the bar.

ii. Then return to starting position, lightly touching the ground.

iii. Raise the left leg out to the side as high as possible, keeping it as straight as possible, pointing your toe without leaning your weight on the bar.

iv. Return to starting position and repeat.

v.   After you have completed all of your repetitions with your left leg, switch legs and repeat with your right leg while holding the aerobic toning bar with your left hand.

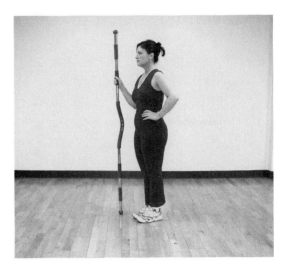

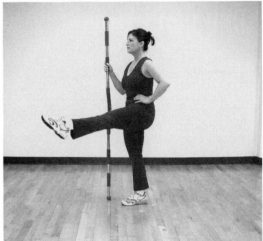

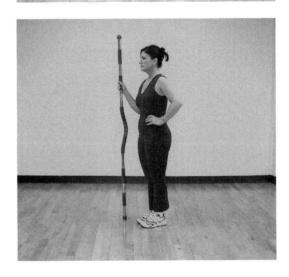

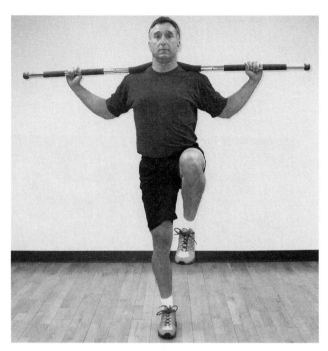

(c) MARCH IN PLACE ON TOES—75 reps

i. Rest the aerobic toning bar across your shoulders with feet about shoulder width apart and raise up to your toes.

ii. Raise left knee straight up to at least waist level toward your chest. Keep back straight and abdominals contracted.

iii. Lower left leg to starting position to toes, making sure that your heels do not touch ground throughout entire movement.

iv. Alternate legs through entire exercise.

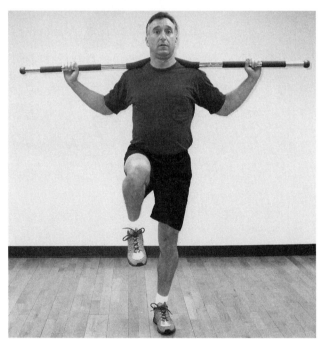

8. Abdominals/Legs: to be performed on a firm exercise mat.

(a) SIT-UPS—50 reps

BEGINNER:

Lie on back with knees bent, feet flat on the floor with heels up against your mat, thumbs clasped, with arms fully extended behind your head. Slowly raise your body all the way up, bringing your chest toward your knees. Exhale while sitting up. Slowly lower body to starting position while inhaling and repeat.

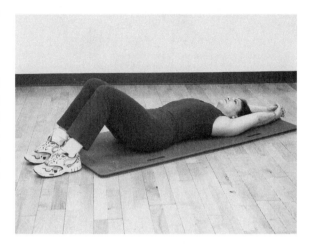

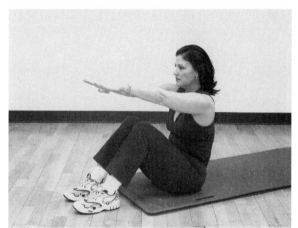

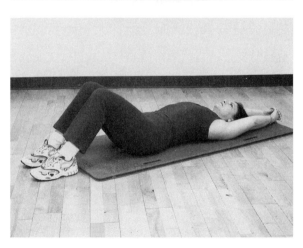

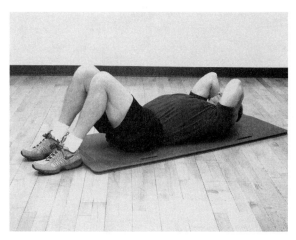

ADVANCED:
Lie on back with knees bent, feet flat on the floor with heels up against your mat, hands on your temples, palms facing in. Slowly raise your body all the way up, bringing your elbows toward your knees. Exhale while sitting up. Slowly lower body to starting position while inhaling and repeat.

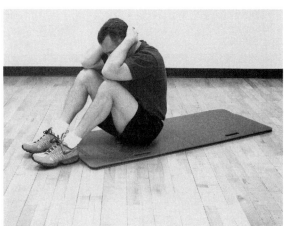

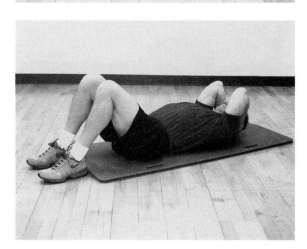

(b) LEG-OUTS—40 to 50 reps

Lying on your back, with hands under buttocks, palms down, bring both knees in toward your chest. Slowly straighten legs out with toes pointed and repeat. Inhale while bringing knees toward chest; exhale as you straighten legs. Beginners should straighten legs out at a higher angle. As you get stronger, try to bring legs lower to the ground (about two inches as illustrated) while straightening legs.

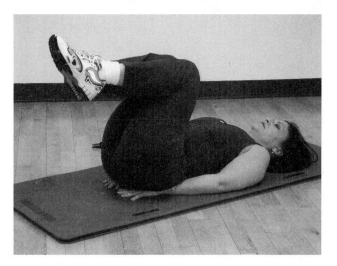

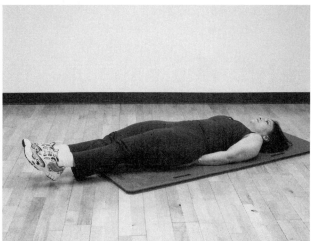

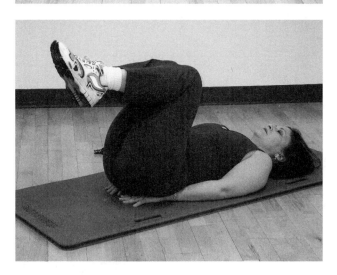

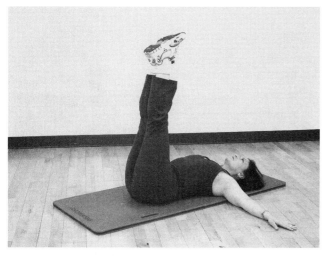

(c) V-SCISSORS (Women only)—40 reps

Lie on your back, hands at your side or with hands under your buttocks with palms facing down. Raise both legs to 90 degrees. Pressing your back into the floor and with toes pointed and legs straight, slowly open legs as far as possible while exhaling. Bring legs back together, keeping toes pointed and legs straight as you inhale and repeat.

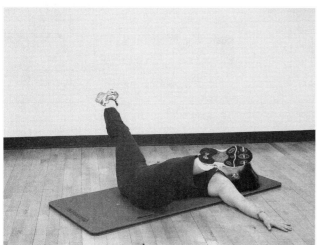

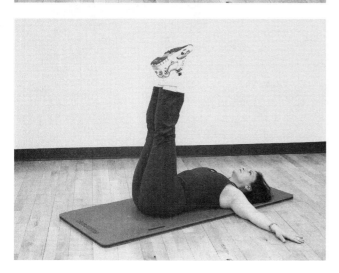

(d) ALTERNATES—60 reps

Lie on your back with your hands under your buttocks or clasped behind your neck with palms down, legs straight and toes pointed. Raise your right leg to a 90-degree angle, your left leg remaining near the floor. Pressing the small of your back into the floor, lower your right leg as you simultaneously lift your left leg to 90 degrees. Repeat this continuous scissoring motion.

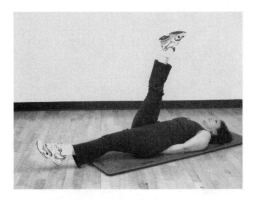

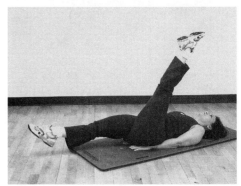

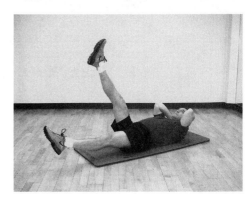

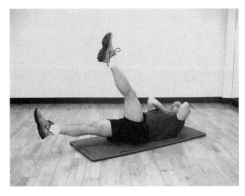

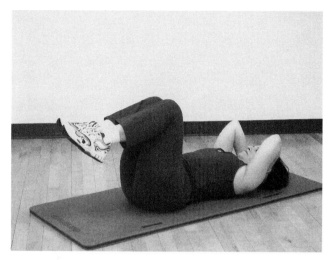

(e) ELBOWS TO KNEES—35 reps

Lying on back, raise knees and feet toward chest in a tucked position. Clasp your hands at the base of your neck. Gently curl your upper body, bringing your elbows toward knees while exhaling. Slowly lower back and shoulders to mat while inhaling and repeat. Keep lower half of your body motionless.

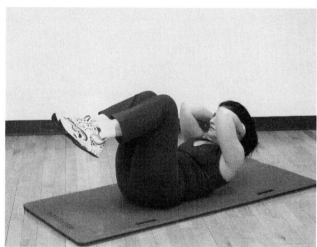

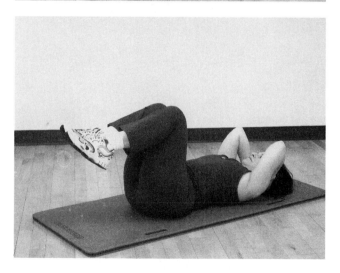

(f) KNEES TO ELBOWS—35 reps

Lying on your back, with hands clasped at the base of your neck, raise head and shoulders slightly off the ground. Raise knees and feet in a tucked position toward elbows, keeping lower back pressed to the floor. Keeping tucked, lower your toes to the ground and repeat. Exhale as you raise knees to elbows; inhale as you lower toes to ground.

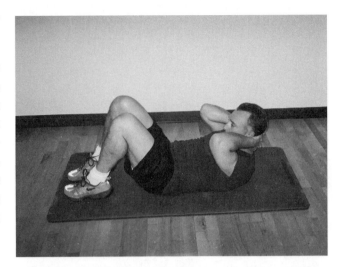

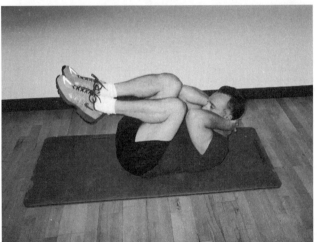

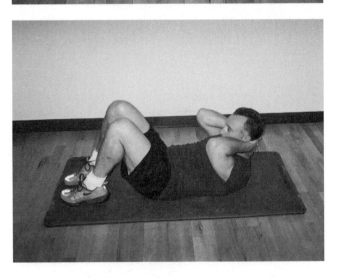

(g) REPEAT SIT-UPS—25 reps

BEGINNER:

ADVANCED:

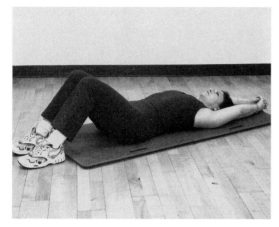

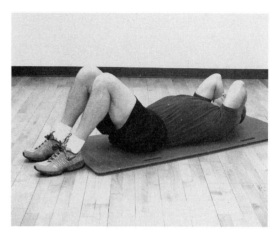

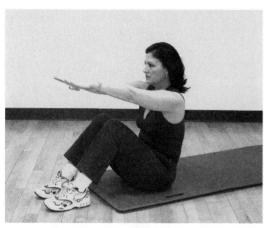

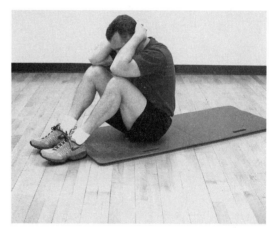

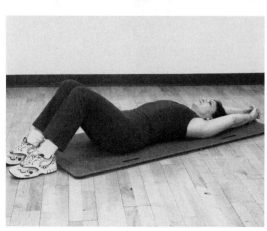

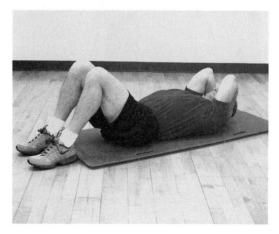

9. **Fat Burner**—jump rope for 5–10 minutes or bike or perform any other aerobic activity of your choice for 10 minutes, vigorously!

JUMP ROPE—5 to 10 MINUTES

OR 10 MINUTES OF AEROBIC EXERCISE

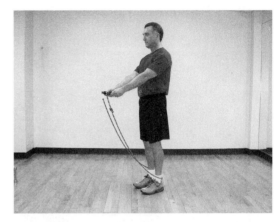

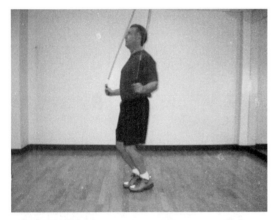

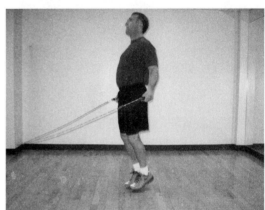

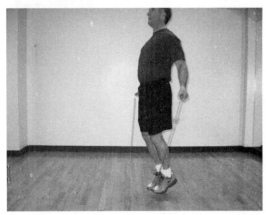

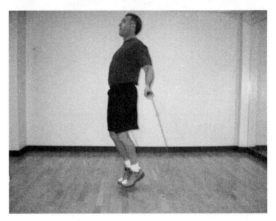

10. **Cooldown**—3 minutes of biking or walking leisurely.

Workout #2—see page 178 for Off Day Routine prescription.

CHAPTER EIGHT

Plans for Losing Those Last 10 Pounds

Most Important Factor in Diet Plans

This is one of the toughest places to lose weight. When you have more weight to lose you have more room to err. When you are down to the last 10 pounds, every little morsel you put in your mouth counts! In this category, one night of extravagant eating can counteract a week's worth of good habits. The most important thing is to stay focused and keep your eye on the goal.

Each time you are challenged and an eating situation comes ups, ask yourself, "Do I want to lose these last few pounds?" Sometimes you really want that treat and that is OK, but the more often you choose not to overeat, the closer you will come to reaching your goals. It is a good idea to take out an outfit, a pair of slacks or jeans, or a suit from your closet that is a little snug and try it on once a week to help keep you motivated and on track. It is also a good idea to keep a food journal to track everything you eat. . . . Often when those last few pounds are not coming off, it is because you are snacking little things here and there that add up without your even realizing it. Remember, it's all about thinking inside the box, and focus, focus, focus!

Helpful Tips for Successful Weight Reduction:

Keep a Food Journal—Write down what and when you eat and drink in a day and why: The journal will help you become aware of what you eat, will increase your control over eating, and will help you become aware of your eating patterns. Food becomes fattening when it is eaten for entertainment, comfort, or stress reduction.

Become Aware of Meal Timing: Eating earlier in the day prevents you from getting too hungry, losing control, and overeating in the evening.

Learn Your Calorie Budget: Know how much you can eat and still lose weight so you can be sure to fuel your body with an adequate amount of essential nutrients.

Eat Slowly: The brain needs about 20 minutes to receive the signal that you've eaten your fill. Practice by putting your fork down between bites and taking pauses throughout the meal.

Keep Away from Food Sources That Tempt You: Out of sight, out of mind, out of **mouth!** Hide high-calorie foods and keep healthy snacks readily available.

Taste Your Food: Calories should be tasted, not wasted. Do nothing else while eating and really savor your food.

Stick to Your Shopping List: Always bring a food list when grocery shopping and never shop while hungry!

Buy Individually Wrapped Packages: Buy your favorite snack foods in individual serving sizes to avoid overeating and further temptation.

Set Realistic Goals: Weight loss greater than 1 percent of your body weight for over two weeks can be dangerous. . . . You can lose muscle, including cardiac muscle. Aim to lose .5–2 pounds per week to ensure you are losing body fat.

Hidden Calorie Foods/Foods to Avoid

- Movie theater popcorn—large with butter contains 1640 calories and 126 gm fat (73 gm saturated!)

- Prime Rib—16 oz. contains 1280 calories and 94 gm fat (52 gm saturated)

- Cheese—1 oz. contains 100 calories and 9 gm fat (6 gm saturated)

- Pizza—Domino's Hand Tossed Cheese (1/8 pie) contains 250 calories and 7 gm fat (4 gm saturated)

- General Tso's chicken—1600 calories and 59 gm fat (11 gm saturated)

- Hamburgers—6-oz. burger on a bun contains 660 calories and 36 gm fat (17 gm saturated)

- Doughnuts—an old-fashioned cake doughnut contains 250 calories and 15 gm fat (3 gm saturated)

- Cinnamon rolls—670 calories and 34 gm fat (14 gm saturated)

- Croissants—5-oz. almond croissant contains 630 calories and 42 gm fat (18 gm saturated)

- French fries—large order contains 500 calories and 28 gm fat (13 gm saturated)

- Tortilla chips—typical basket (51 chips) contains 640 calories and 34 gm fat (6 gm saturated)

- Grilled cheese sandwich—500 calories and 33 gm fat (17 gm saturated)

- Fettuccine alfredo—1500 calories and 97 gm fat (48 gm saturated)

- Starbucks white chocolate mocha (made with whole milk)—600 calories and 25 gm fat (15 gm saturated)

- Pancakes with syrup and margarine (3 pancakes with 1/4 cup syrup and 1 tbsp. margarine)—770 calories and 22 gm fat (9 gm saturated)

*Please note: For those individuals who are vegetarian or have other special dietary needs, please log on to eatright.org or ediets.com to find a dietician near you.

Meal Plans for Losing Those Last 10 Pounds

Limited Approach
1200 CALORIES, PER DAY
(165 GM CARBOHYDRATE, 60 GM PROTEIN, 33 GM FAT)

BREAKFAST *(400 calories, approx. 55 gm carbohydrate, 20 gm protein, 11 gm fat):*

1. (400 calories, 57 gm carb, 14 gm protein, 10 gm fat)

   1 1/2 cups whole grain cereal (unsweetened, ready-to-eat cereal)

   1 cup skim milk

   1 cup berries

   12 almonds

2. (400 calories, 45 gm carb, 20 gm protein, 12 gm fat)

   $^1/_2$ cup 1 percent cottage cheese

   1 cup berries

   12 almonds

   2 slices of whole grain bread

3. (400 calories, 55 gm carb, 18 gm protein, 8 gm fat)

   2 slices of whole grain bread

   1 tbsp. peanut butter

   1 apple

   6 oz. low-fat yogurt

4. (400 calories, 53 gm carb, 20 gm protein, 10 gm fat)

   2 poached eggs

   2 slices of whole grain bread

   1 $^1/_2$ cups melon

5. (400 calories, 48 gm carb, 20 gm protein, 11 gm fat)

   1 cup cooked oatmeal

   9 chopped walnut halves

   1 chopped Red Delicious apple

   $^1/_2$ cup low-fat cottage cheese

6. (400 calories, 45 gm carb, 23 gm protein, 10 gm fat)

   Omelet—1 whole egg and 2 egg whites + $^1/_2$ ounce of low-fat cheese + $^1/_2$ cup spinach

   2 slices of whole grain bread

   1 cup sliced strawberries

7. (400 calories, 50 gm carb, 19 gm protein, 10 gm fat)

   2 slices of whole grain bread

   1 $^1/_2$ oz. cheese

   $^1/_2$ cup sliced tomato

   1 cup mixed melon

LUNCH (400 calories, approx. 55 gm carbohydrate, 20 gm protein, 11 gm fat):

1. (400 calories, 50 gm carb, 22 gm protein, 10 gm fat)

   2 slices of whole grain bread

   2 oz. white meat turkey

   $^1/_4$ avocado

   $^1/_2$ cup sliced tomato and lettuce

   1 medium apple

2. (400 calories, 50 gm carb, 22 gm protein, 10 gm fat)

   1 whole wheat pita

   2 oz. chunk white tuna fish

   2 tsps. mayonnaise

   $^1/_2$ cup mixed shredded carrots, lettuce, and celery

   1 medium orange

3. (400 calories, 50 gm carb, 22 gm protein, 10 gm fat)

   2 oz. cold chicken (cut up), mixed with 2 tsps. mayonnaise

   2 slices of rye bread

   $^1/_2$ cup sliced tomato and lettuce

   $^1/_2$ diced mango

4. (400 calories, 50 gm carb, 25 gm protein, 10 gm fat)

   Big Salad:

   > 2 cups mixed greens
   >
   > 1/2 cup diced carrots
   >
   > 1/2 cup diced bell peppers
   >
   > 1/3 cup beans
   >
   > 2 oz. grilled chicken
   >
   > 2 tbsps. vinaigrette salad dressing
   >
   > 1 medium nectarine

5. (400 calories, 55 gm carb, 24 gm protein, 10 gm fat)

   > 2 oz. lean roast beef
   >
   > 2 slices rye bread
   >
   > 1 tsp. mayonnaise
   >
   > 1/2 cup sliced tomato and lettuce
   >
   > 1/2 cup carrot sticks
   >
   > 3/4 cup fresh pineapple

6. (400 calories, 45 gm carb, 25 gm protein, 15 gm fat)

   > 2 cups spinach
   >
   > 1 oz. feta cheese
   >
   > 1 oz. firm tofu
   >
   > 1/2 cup water chestnuts
   >
   > 1/2 cup snap peas
   >
   > 3/4 cup mandarin oranges
   >
   > 1 tbsp. reduced-fat ginger salad dressing
   >
   > 5 whole grain crackers

7. (400 calories, 50 gm carb, 21 gm protein, 10 gm fat)

   > 2 slices of whole grain bread
   >
   > 1 oz. white meat turkey
   >
   > 1 oz. low-fat cheese
   >
   > 1 tsp. mayonnaise
   >
   > 1/2 cup sliced tomato and lettuce
   >
   > 2 small plums

DINNER *(400 calories, approx. 55 gm carbohydrate, 20 gm protein, 11 gm fat):*

1. (400 calories, 50 gm carb, 26 gm protein, 10 gm fat)

   > 2 oz. cooked chicken (no skin)
   >
   > 2/3 cup brown rice
   >
   > 1/2 cup green beans sautéed in 1 tsp. olive oil
   >
   > 1 cup mixed greens with 1/2 cup chopped tomatoes and 1/2 cup chopped peppers
   >
   > 1 tbsp. salad dressing

2. (400 calories, 55 gm carb, 24 gm protein, 11 gm fat)

   > 2 oz. lean cooked roast beef
   >
   > 1/2 cup carrots

   > 1/2 cup cauliflower
   >
   > 1 tsp. olive oil
   >
   > 1 whole grain dinner roll
   >
   > 1 orange

3. (400 calories, 48 gm carb, 24 gm protein, 11 gm fat)

   > 2 oz. broiled salmon
   >
   > 1 medium sweet potato
   >
   > 1 cup sautéed spinach with 1 tsp. olive oil
   >
   > 1/2 cup sliced tomato
   >
   > 1/2 cup diced melon

4. (400 calories, 50 gm carb, 25 gm protein, 10 gm fat)

    2 oz. sautéed shrimp in 1 tsp. olive oil

    1 cup whole wheat pasta

    1/2 cup jarred tomato sauce

    1/2 cup artichoke hearts

5. (400 calories, 50 gm carb, 22 gm protein, 10 gm fat)

    2 oz. baked cod

    2 cups baked winter squash

    1 cup mixed greens (kale, collard, and mustard) sautéed in 2 tsps. olive oil

    1 cup cubed papaya

6. (400 calories, 48 gm carb, 24 gm protein, 11 gm fat)

    2 oz. flank steak

    2/3 cup whole wheat couscous

    2 cups roasted broccoli and cauliflower with 1 tsp. olive oil

    1/2 cup raspberries

7. (400 calories, 48 gm carb, 24 gm protein, 11 gm fat)

    2 oz. barbecued chicken

    1 medium corn on the cob

    1/3 cup baked beans

    1 cup cucumber and tomato salad tossed with 1 tbsp. olive oil–based dressing

    1/2 cup cubed watermelon

Dynamic Approach
1600 CALORIES PER DAY
(221 GM CARBOHYDRATE, 80 GM PROTEIN, 44 GM FAT)

BREAKFAST *(400 calories, approx. 55 gm carbohydrate, 20 gm protein, 11 gm fat):*

1. (400 calories, 57 gm carb, 14 gm protein, 10 gm fat)

    1 1/2 cups whole grain cereal (unsweetened, ready-to-eat cereal)

    1 cup skim milk

    1 cup berries

    12 almonds

2. (400 calories, 45 gm carb, 20 gm protein, 12 gm fat)

    1/2 cup 1 percent cottage cheese

    1 cup berries

    12 almonds

    2 slices of whole grain bread

3. (400 calories, 55 gm carb, 18 gm protein, 8 gm fat)

    2 slices of whole grain bread

    1 tbsp. peanut butter

    1 apple

    6 oz. low-fat yogurt

4. (400 calories, 53 gm carb, 20 gm protein, 10 gm fat)

    2 poached eggs

2 slices of whole grain bread

1 ¹/₂ cups melon

5. (400 calories, 48 gm carb, 20 gm protein, 11 gm fat)

   1 cup cooked oatmeal

   9 chopped walnut halves

   1 chopped Red Delicious apple

   ¹/₂ cup low-fat cottage cheese

6. (400 calories, 45 gm carb, 23 gm protein, 10 gm fat)

   Omelet—1 whole egg and 2 egg whites + ¹/₂ oz. of low-fat cheese + ¹/₂ cup spinach

2 slices of whole grain bread

cup sliced strawberries

7. (400 calories, 50 gm carb, 19 gm protein, 10 gm fat)

   2 slices of whole grain bread

   1 ¹/₂ oz. cheese

   ¹/₂ cup sliced tomato

   1 cup mixed melon

LUNCH *(500 calories, approx. 68 gm carbohydrate, 25 gm protein, 14 gm fat):*

1. (500 calories, 65 gm carb, 22 gm protein, 15 gm fat)

   2 slices of whole grain bread

   2 oz. white meat turkey

   ¹/₄ avocado

   ¹/₂ cup sliced tomato and lettuce

   ¹/₂ cup unsweetened apple sauce with ¹/₄ cup low-fat granola

2. (500 calories, 65 gm carb, 22 gm protein, 15 gm fat)

   1 whole wheat pita

   2 oz. chunk white tuna fish

   3 tsps. mayonnaise

   ¹/₂ cup mixed shredded carrots, lettuce, and celery

   24 cherries

3. (500 calories, 65 gm carb, 22 gm protein, 15 gm fat)

   2 oz. cold chicken (cut up) mixed with 3 tsps. mayonnaise

   2 slices of rye bread

   ¹/₂ cup sliced tomato and lettuce

   1 whole diced mango

4. (500 calories, 65 gm carb, 25 gm protein, 15 gm fat)

   Big Salad:

   2 cups mixed greens

   ¹/₂ cup diced carrots

   ¹/₂ cup diced bell peppers

   ¹/₃ cup beans

   2 oz. grilled chicken

   4 chopped walnuts

1 diced apple

2 tbsps. vinaigrette salad dressing

1 medium nectarine

5. (500 calories, 70 gm carb, 24 gm protein, 15 gm fat)

2 oz. lean roast beef

2 slices of rye bread

1 tsp. mayonnaise

1/2 cup sliced tomato and lettuce

1/2 cup carrot sticks

1 1/2 cup fresh pineapple topped with 6 slivered almonds

6. (500 calories, 60 gm carb, 28 gm protein, 15 gm fat)

2 cups spinach

1 oz. feta cheese

1 oz. firm tofu

1/2 cup water chestnuts

1/2 cup snap peas

3/4 cup mandarin oranges

1 tbsp. reduced-fat ginger salad dressing

10 whole grain crackers

7. (500 calories, 65 gm carb, 28 gm protein, 15 gm fat)

2 slices of whole grain bread

2 oz. white meat turkey

1 oz. low-fat cheese

2 tsps. mayonnaise

1/2 cup sliced tomato and lettuce

1 1/2 cups mixed fruit salad

SNACK *(200 calories, approx. 27 gm carb, 10 gm protein, 6 gm fat):*

1. (200 calories, 27 gm carb, 8 gm protein, 5 gm fat)

1 cup plain nonfat yogurt

3/4 cup fresh blackberries

6 chopped almonds

2. (200 calories, 27 gm carb, 8 gm protein, 5 gm fat)

1 medium apple

2 tsps. peanut butter

1 cup skim milk

3. (200 calories, 30 gm carb, 7 gm protein, 7 gm fat)

1 whole grain English muffin

1 oz. Swiss cheese

4. (200 calories, 27 gm carb, 8 gm protein, 5 gm fat)

PB&J smoothie:

Blend 1 cup skim + 1 1/4 cups fresh or frozen strawberries + 2 tsps. peanut butter

5. (200 calories, 27 gm carb, 8 gm protein, 5 gm fat)

six-inch whole wheat pita

1 sliced apple

2 tsps. peanut butter

6. (200 calories, 27 gm carb, 8 gm protein, 5 gm fat)

1 slice whole wheat raisin bread topped with 1 sliced kiwi and 1/4 cup ricotta cheese

7. (200 calories, 27 gm carb, 8 gm protein, 5 gm fat)

   1/2 six-inch whole wheat pita

   1/3 cup hummus

   1/2 cup carrot sticks

DINNER *(500 calories, approx. 68 gm carbohydrate, 25 gm protein, 14 gm fat):*

1. (500 calories, 65 gm carb, 26 gm protein, 15 gm fat)

   2 oz. cooked chicken (no skin)

   2/3 cup brown rice

   1/2 cup green beans sautéed in 1 tsp. olive oil and 6 slivered almonds

   1 cup mixed greens with 1/2 cup chopped tomatoes and 1/2 cup chopped peppers

   1 tbsp. salad dressing

   1 medium apple

2. (500 calories, 70 gm carb, 23 gm protein, 14 gm fat)

   2 oz. lean cooked roast beef

   1/3 cup brown rice

   1/2 cup carrots

   1/2 cup cauliflower

   1 1/2 tsps. olive oil

   1 whole grain dinner roll

   1 orange

3. (500 calories, 68 gm carb, 29 gm protein, 14 gm fat)

   2 oz. broiled salmon

   1 large sweet potato

   1 cup sautéed spinach with 1 1/2 tsp. olive oil

   1 cup sliced tomato

   1/2 cup diced melon

4. (500 calories, 50 gm carb, 25 gm protein, 14 gm fat)

   2 oz. sautéed shrimp in 1 1/2 tsps. olive oil

   1 cup whole wheat pasta

   1/2 cup jarred tomato sauce

   1/2 cup artichoke hearts

   1 1/4 cups sliced strawberries

5. (500 calories, 65 gm carb, 29 gm protein, 14 gm fat)

   3 oz. baked cod

   2 cups baked winter squash

   1 cup mixed greens (kale, collard, and mustard) sautéed in 2 1/2 tsps. olive oil

   2 cups cubed papaya

6. (500 calories, 70 gm carb, 27 gm protein, 14 gm fat)

   2 oz. flank steak

   1 cup whole wheat couscous

   2 cups roasted broccoli and cauliflower with 1 1/2 tsps. olive oil

   3/4 cup raspberries

7. (500 calories, 68 gm carb, 27 gm protein, 14 gm fat)

   2 oz. barbecued chicken

   1 medium corn on the cob

   2/3 cup baked beans

   1 1/2 cups cucumber and tomato salad tossed with 1 1/2 tbsps. olive oil–based dressing

   1/2 cup cubed watermelon

Balanced Approach

1400 CALORIES PER DAY

(192 GM CARBOHYDRATE, 70 GM PROTEIN, 39 GM FAT)

BREAKFAST *(400 calories, approx. 55 gm carbohydrate, 20 gm protein, 11 gm fat):*

1. (400 calories, 57 gm carb, 14 gm protein, 10 gm fat)

    1 1/2 cups whole grain cereal (unsweetened, ready-to-eat cereal)

    1 cup skim milk

    1 cup berries

    12 almonds

2. (400 calories, 45 gm carb, 20 gm protein, 12 gm fat)

    1/2 cup 1 percent cottage cheese

    1 cup berries

    12 almonds

    2 slices of whole grain bread

3. (400 calories, 55 gm carb, 18 gm protein, 8 gm fat)

    2 slices of whole grain bread

    1 tbsp. peanut butter

    1 apple

    6 oz. low-fat yogurt

4. (400 calories, 53 gm carb, 20 gm protein, 10 gm fat)

    2 poached eggs

    2 slices of whole grain bread

    1 1/2 cups melon

5. (400 calories, 48 gm carb, 20 gm protein, 11 gm fat)

    1 cup cooked oatmeal

    9 chopped walnut halves

    1 chopped Red Delicious apple

    1/2 cup low-fat cottage cheese

6. (400 calories, 45 gm carb, 23 gm protein, 10 gm fat)

    Omelet—1 whole egg and 2 egg whites + 1/2 ounce of low-fat cheese + 1/2 cup spinach

    2 slices of whole grain bread

    1 cup sliced strawberries

7. (400 calories, 50 gm carb, 19 gm protein, 11 gm fat)

    2 slices of whole grain bread

    1 1/2 oz. cheese

    1/2 cup sliced tomato

    1 cup mixed melon

LUNCH *(400 calories, approx. 55 gm carbohydrate, 20 gm protein, 11 gm fat):*

1. (400 calories, 50 gm carb, 22 gm protein, 10 gm fat)

   2 slices of whole grain bread

   2 oz. white meat turkey

   1/4 avocado

   1/2 cup sliced tomato and lettuce

   1 medium apple

2. (400 calories, 50 gm carb, 22 gm protein, 10 gm fat)

   1 whole wheat pita

   2 oz. chunk white tuna fish

   2 tsps. mayonnaise

   1/2 cup mixed shredded carrots, lettuce, and celery

   1 medium orange

3. (400 calories, 50 gm carb, 22 gm protein, 10 gm fat)

   2 oz. cold chicken (cut up) mixed with 2 tsps. mayonnaise

   2 slices of rye bread

   1/2 cup sliced tomato and lettuce

   1/2 diced mango

4. (400 calories, 50 gm carb, 25 gm protein, 10 gm fat)

   Big Salad:

       2 cups mixed greens

       1/2 cup diced carrots

       1/2 cup diced bell peppers

       1/3 cup beans

       2 oz. grilled chicken

       2 tbsp. vinaigrette salad dressing

   1 medium nectarine

5. (400 calories, 55 gm carb, 24 gm protein, 10 gm fat)

   2 oz. lean roast beef

   2 slices of rye bread

   1 tsp. mayonnaise

   1/2 cup sliced tomato and lettuce

   1/2 cup carrot sticks

   3/4 cup fresh pineapple

6. (400 calories, 45 gm carb, 25 gm protein, 15 gm fat)

   2 cups spinach

   1 oz. feta cheese

   1 oz. firm tofu

   1/2 cup water chestnuts

   1/2 cup snap peas

   3/4 cup mandarin oranges

   1 tbsp. reduced-fat ginger salad dressing

   5 whole grain crackers

7. (400 calories, 50 gm carb, 21 gm protein, 10 gm fat)

   2 slices of whole grain bread

   1 oz. white meat turkey

   1 oz. low-fat cheese

   1 tsp. mayonnaise

   1/2 cup sliced tomato and lettuce

   2 small plums

SNACK *(200 calories, approx. 27 gm carb, 10 gm protein, 6 gm fat):*

1. (200 calories, 27 gm carb, 8 gm protein, 5 gm fat)

   1 cup plain nonfat yogurt

   $^3/_4$ cup fresh blackberries

   6 chopped almonds

2. (200 calories, 27 gm carb, 8 gm protein, 5 gm fat)

   1 medium apple

   2 tsps. peanut butter

   1 cup skim milk

3. (200 calories, 30 gm carb, 7 gm protein, 7 gm fat)

   1 whole grain English muffin

   1 oz. Swiss cheese

4. (200 calories, 27 gm carb, 8 gm protein, 5 gm fat)

   PB&J smoothie:

   > Blend 1 cup skim + 1 $^1/_4$ cups fresh or frozen strawberries + 2 tsps. peanut butter

5. (200 calories, 27 gm carb, 8 gm protein, 5 gm fat)

   six-inch whole wheat pita

   1 sliced apple

   2 tsps. peanut butter

6. (200 calories, 27 gm carb, 8 gm protein, 5 gm fat)

   1 slice whole wheat raisin bread topped with 1 sliced kiwi and $^1/_4$ cup ricotta cheese

7. (200 calories, 27 gm carb, 8 gm protein, 5 gm fat)

   $^1/_2$ six-inch whole wheat pita

   $^1/_3$ cup hummus

   $^1/_2$ cup carrot sticks

DINNER *(400 calories, approx. 55 gm carbohydrate, 20 gm protein, 11 gm fat):*

1. (400 calories, 50 gm carb, 26 gm protein, 10 gm fat)

   2 oz. cooked chicken (no skin)

   $^2/_3$ cup brown rice

   $^1/_2$ cup green beans sautéed in 1 tsp. olive oil

   1 cup mixed greens with $^1/_2$ cup chopped tomatoes and $^1/_2$ cup chopped peppers

   1 tbsp. salad dressing

2. (400 calories, 55 gm carb, 24 gm protein, 11 gm fat)

   2 oz. lean cooked roast beef

   $^1/_2$ cup carrots

   $^1/_2$ cup cauliflower

   1 tsp. olive oil

   1 whole grain dinner roll

   1 orange

3. (400 calories, 48 gm carb, 24 gm protein, 11 gm fat)

   2 oz. broiled salmon

   1 medium sweet potato

   1 cup sautéed spinach with 1 tsp. olive oil

   1/2 cup sliced tomato

   1/2 cup diced melon

4. (400 calories, 50 gm carb, 25 gm protein, 10 gm fat)

   2 oz. sautéed shrimp in 1 tsp. olive oil

   1 cup whole wheat pasta

   1/2 cup jarred tomato sauce

   1/2 cup artichoke hearts

5. (400 calories, 50 gm carb, 22 gm protein, 10 gm fat)

   2 oz. baked cod

   2 cups baked winter squash

   1 cup mixed greens (kale, collard, and mustard) sautéed in 2 tsps. olive oil

   1 cup cubed papaya

6. (400 calories, 48 gm carb, 24 gm protein, 11 gm fat)

   2 oz. flank steak

   2/3 cup whole wheat couscous

   2 cups roasted broccoli and cauliflower with 1 tsp. olive oil

   1/2 cup raspberries

7. (400 calories, 48 gm carb, 24 gm protein, 11 gm fat)

   2 oz. barbecued chicken

   1 medium corn on the cob

   1/3 cup baked beans

   1 cup cucumber and tomato salad tossed with 1 tbsp. olive oil–based dressing

   1/2 cup cubed watermelon

Additional Foods to Choose as Between Meal Snacks

LOW-CALORIE

Fresh fruit

Fresh vegetables (can dip them in 2 tbsps. hummus, salsa, or homemade low-fat dip)

Low-fat yogurt

Low-fat cottage cheese

Hot-air-popped popcorn

MEDIUM-CALORIE

1/4 cup dry-roasted nuts (need to limit portions)

1 tbsp. nut butter on a slice of whole wheat bread

1 tbsp. nut butter on a medium apple

2 tsps. peanut butter + 2 graham crackers + 2 tsps. jam

1 oz. of reduced-fat cheese with 10 whole grain crackers

1 slice of reduced-fat cheese melted over tomato on whole grain bread

Nonfat Greek yogurt with 1 cup of berries and 2 tbsps. chopped nuts

1/4 cup dry roasted mixed nuts (almonds, pumpkinseeds, walnuts)

1/2 whole wheat English muffin + 1 slice low-fat mozzarella cheese + 1 tbsp. marinara sauce

1 medium orange diced into 1 serving of oatmeal + 2 walnut halves

FOR SWEET CRAVINGS

Fresh watermelon

Fresh berries

Sugar-free Jell-O

Fat-free/sugar-free fudge pop

Sugar-free Popsicle

FOR SAVORY CRAVINGS

Fresh vegetables dipped in salsa

Hot-air-popped popcorn

Exercise Prescription for Losing Those Last 10 Pounds

Most Important Factor

This is the toughest amount of weight to get off because when most people get this close, there isn't as much urgency or social, family, or peer pressure to lose weight. You must decrease your diet significantly, meaning the total calories you consume, as well as exercise with high intensity in order to shed these final pounds. It is vital that you carefully monitor what you're eating and drinking, because "hidden" calories plus the fact that most people eat a little more than usual because they feel they are allowed due to their workouts, are usually the reasons most individuals do not reach their goals at this critical juncture.

Fitness Equipment Needed

1. **Choose One:** Recumbent or upright stationary bike, treadmill, elliptical machine or cross trainer or, if no access to any equipment, jog/run instead

2. Firm exercise mat

3. A lightweight (2–4 lb.) collapsible aerobic toning bar for both men and women

4. A 10-lb. weight bar for women, 15-lb. weight bar for men

5. A lightweight speed or beaded jump rope

While jumping rope, make sure you jump on a surface that has a give to it, such as a wooden floor, short grass, a rubberized track or tennis court, or the like. *Do not* jump on asphalt or cement. If you don't have access to this type of surface and/or need help in improving your jump rope skills, log onto *www.exude.com* to view Jump Rope Mat and Jumping Toward Fitness Video.

Please Note: All of the following exercise regimens can be performed at home, at the gym, or even while traveling.

Exercise Regimen

Frequency—3, 4, or 5 days per week

Duration—60 to 75 minutes, depending upon your current level of fitness

**Before starting this or any exercise regimen, get your doctor's approval.

Workout #1

Full-Body Routine—3 days per week, every other day, Mondays, Wednesdays, and Fridays or Tuesdays, Thursdays, and Saturdays.

"**Reps**" = Repetitions, the number of times you actually perform the exercise.

1. **Warm-up**—20 minutes of biking with moderate tension at 100 + RPMs, fast walk at 4.5 MPH, jog/run at 6.0 + MPH, elliptical or cross trainer—vigorously!

2. **Stretch**—3 minutes.

3. **Fat Burner**—7 minutes of jumping rope, or 3 minutes of marching in place on toes, then 4 minutes of favorite aerobic piece of equipment of your choice, vigorously!

4. **Chest/Arms**—(a) push-ups: 10 to 25 reps, then 50 side benders; (b) repeat push-ups 10 to 25 reps.

5. **Abdominals/Legs**—(a) sit-ups: 75 reps; (b) leg lifts: 25 reps, rest 10 seconds, then repeat 25 reps; (c) leg-outs: 60 reps; (d) V-scissors: 50 to 60 reps; (e) alternates: 75 to 100 reps; (f) elbows to knees: 40 reps; (g) knees to elbows: 40 reps.

6. **Legs/buttocks**—(a) squat thrusts: 20 to 30 reps; (b) lunges with aerobic or weighted bar: 20 to 30 reps; (c) dead lifts with aerobic or weighted bar: 40 to 50 reps.

7. **Legs/Hips**—(a) standing knee to opposite chest: 50 reps each leg; (b) march in place on toes: 100 reps.

8. **Upper Body Exercise**—with weighted bar: (a) push-outs: 30 reps; (b) behind the neck press: 30 reps; (c) front press: 30 reps; (d) wide upright rows: 30 reps; (e) narrow upright rows: 30 reps; (f) curls: 30 reps; (g) kick backs: 30 reps; (h) advanced kick-backs: 20 reps.

9. **Legs/Buttocks**—(a) squat thrusts: 20 reps; (b) lunges: 20 reps; (c) dead lifts: 40 reps.

10. **Fat Burner**—7 minutes of jumping rope or 3 minutes of marching in place on toes, then 4 minutes of favorite aerobic piece of equipment of your choice, vigorously!

11. **Cooldown**—3 minutes of walking or biking leisurely.

___

If you need a break at any time during your exercise regimen, you can simply get on a stationary bike or any other piece of aerobic equipment or walk for a minute or so to allow your heart rate to come down safely *before* you resume. Also, if time allows, do another set of exercises for your upper body, midsection, or lower body if you want to improve that region of your body in a shorter period of time.

One of your goals is to build up to 100 repetitions for all your abdominal exercises and 50–60 repetitions for all upper body exercises. You should be increasing your repetitions on every exercise 1–2 repetitions every 2–3 weeks. Try to work up to 30 minutes of continuous rope jumping without a break, and if you cannot jump rope because of a medical or orthopedic concern, increase the speed and resistance on your favorite piece of aerobic equipment to ensure the proper intensity.

Workout #2 (Optional, depending upon which approach you choose: Balanced or Dynamic)

Off Day Routine—2 to 3 days per week on days in between Full-Body Routines

1. Aerobic exercise of your choice for 50 minutes—vigorously!

2. Stretch 3 minutes.

3. Cooldown—3 minutes of walking or biking leisurely.

___

**Please Note: If you want to and time allows, you may perform any of the abdominal/leg exercises and/or legs/hips exercises only, prior to cooling down.

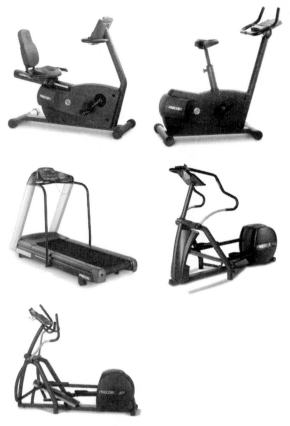

1. Aerobic Equipment

2. Firm Exercise Mat

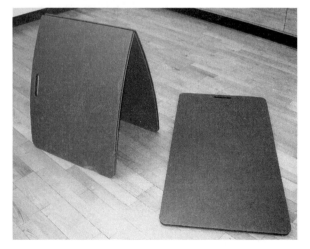

3. Collapsible Aerobic Toning Bar

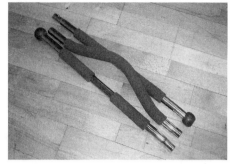

Unassembled

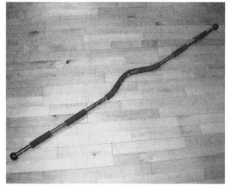

Assembled

4. Weighted Bar

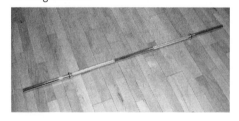

5. Speed and Beaded Jump Rope.

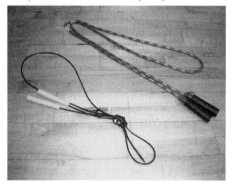

Workout #1—Full-Body Routine

1. Warm-up—20 minutes.

2. Stretch: hold each stretch for 30–60 seconds.

ARM CIRCLES

With arms outstretched, slowly circle your arms backward for 5 revolutions and then forward for 5 revolutions.

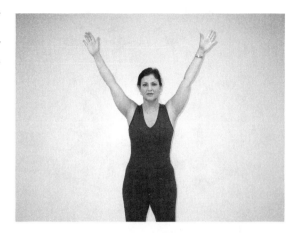

TRICEPS

With arms overhead, gently pull the left elbow behind your head with your right hand. Hold when you reach a comfortable stretch in the rear shoulder and upper back. Switch arms and repeat.

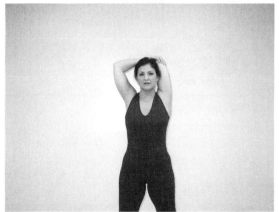

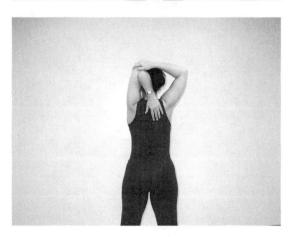

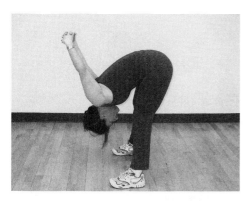

SHOULDERS, CHEST, AND HAMSTRINGS

Grasp hands behind your back, with palms facing each other. Slightly bend your knees and lift arms up as you bend forward at the waist. Hold when you feel a comfortable stretch in the shoulders, chest, and hamstrings.

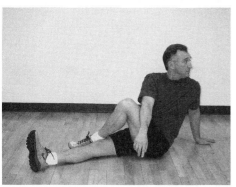

SPINAL TWIST

Keeping the right leg straight, left arm behind for support, cross left leg over and place foot outside the right knee. With the right hand or elbow on the left knee, slowly twist and look over your left shoulder while simultaneously pulling the knee in the opposite direction; hold. You will feel pressure in the hip, side, and upper back. Repeat on opposite side.

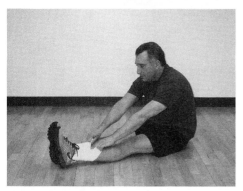

HAMSTRINGS

With legs straight, ankles flexed, bend forward from the hips and reach out toward your toes and, based on your flexibility, grab on to either your socks or shoelaces while holding the stretch. You will feel tension just behind the knees, in your upper calves, and in the lower back area. If possible, you should also perform this stretch with legs apart, using the preceding instructions.

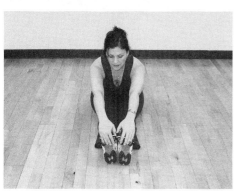

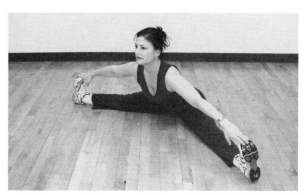

GROIN

In sitting position, pull your soles of your feet together and grab hold of your ankles. Gently pull heels toward the groin area. Let your knees relax toward the floor, and gently press your elbows down on your knees to increase the stretch.

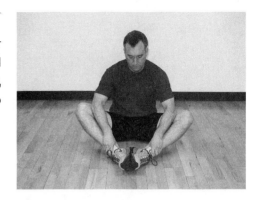

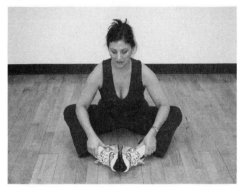

QUADRICEPS

Lie down on your left side. Bend your right leg and grab your right ankle with your hand. Gently pull your right leg back toward your buttocks. Hold the position when you feel a comfortable stretch in front of your right thigh. Release slowly and roll over to your left side and repeat.

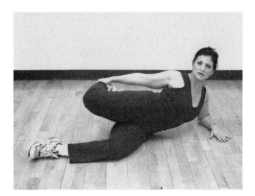

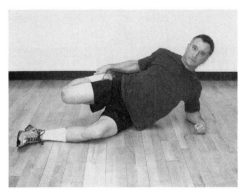

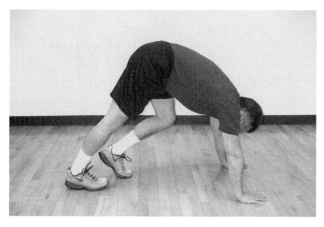

CALVES #1

With hands and knees on all fours, straighten your body into a **V** position. With both feet together, bend your left knee and press your right heel toward the ground, stretching your right calf. Repeat on other side.

OR

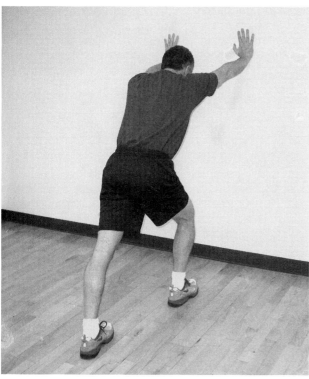

CALVES #2

Stand a little farther than arm's length away from a wall or solid support, lean on it with hands placed shoulder distance away. Bring one foot forward, knee bent, while keeping the back leg straight heel pressing into the floor. Lean toward wall while holding stretch. Switch legs and repeat.

3. **Fat Burner**—7 minutes of jumping rope or 3 minutes of marching in place on toes, then 4 minutes of favorite aerobic piece of equipment of your choice, vigorously!

JUMPING ROPE—7 MINUTES

How to Jump Rope:

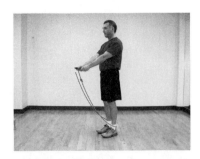

i.   Practice swinging rope over head without jumping, forming a loop.

ii. Move forearms in time with feet.

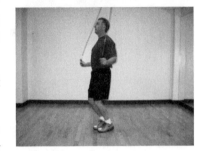

iii. Jump just high enough for rope to pass under feet (one inch off the ground). Jump with both feet at once. (Jumping higher than one inch will create unnecessary stress on the legs, increasing the potential for injury.)

iv. Rope should hit the ground about one foot in front of feet with each revolution.

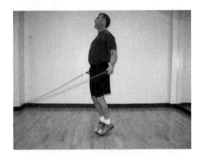

v.   Caution: Avoid double jumping. Your workout will not be as effective! After each jump the rope should pass under your feet.

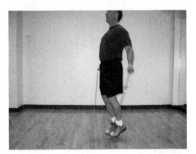

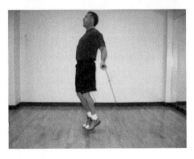

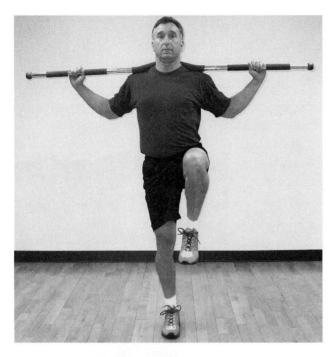

OR MARCH IN PLACE ON TOES—3 MINUTES

i.   Rest the aerobic toning bar across your shoulders with feet about shoulder width apart and rise up to your toes.

ii. Raise left knee straight up to at least waist level toward your chest. Keep back straight and abdominals contracted.

iii. Lower left leg to starting position to toes, making sure that your heels do not touch ground throughout entire movement.

iv. Alternate legs through entire exercise.

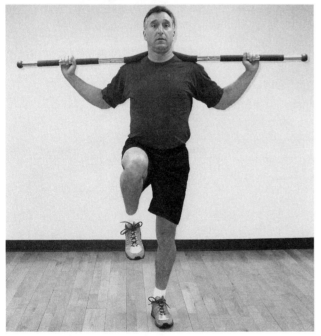

4 MINUTES OF AEROBIC EXERCISE

4. Chest/Arms.

(a) PUSH-UPS—10 to 25 reps

Basic—on hands and knees with ankles crossed, place hands slightly wider than shoulder width apart, arms straight, fingers forward, and abdominals contracted. While inhaling, lower chest as close to the floor as possible. Exhale while pushing up to starting position and repeat. Keep lower body still through entire movement.

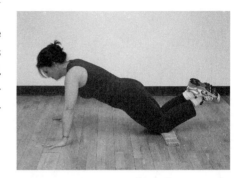

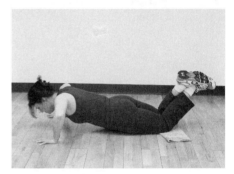

Advanced—extend body on hands and toes with arms straight and place hands slightly wider than shoulder width apart, fingers forward, and abdominals contracted. While inhaling, lower chest as close to the floor as possible. Exhale while pushing up to starting position and repeat. Do not jerk your body or arch your back while performing exercise.

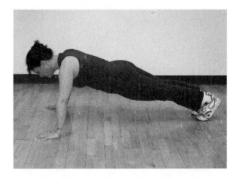

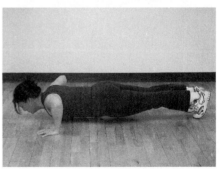

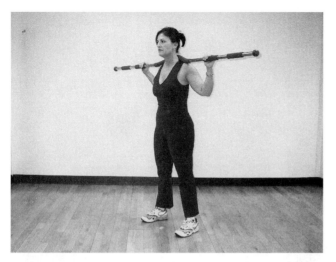

SIDE BENDERS—50 reps

Rest after push-ups by doing side benders until you catch your breath.

i. Rest the aerobic toning bar across your shoulders and slowly bend your upper body from side to side.

ii. Keep your lower body still, moving only at the waist.

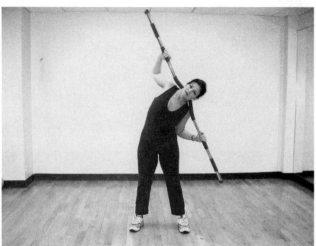

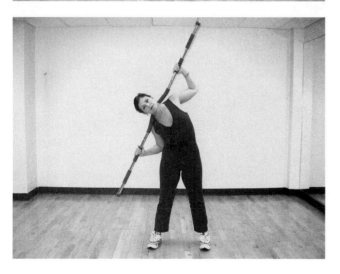

(b) Repeat PUSH-UPS—10 to 25 reps

Basic

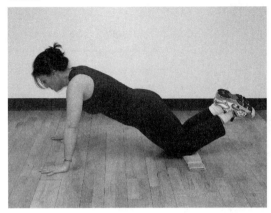 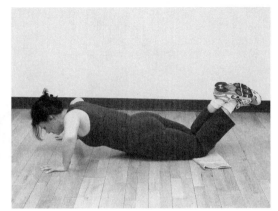

Advanced

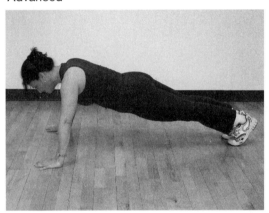 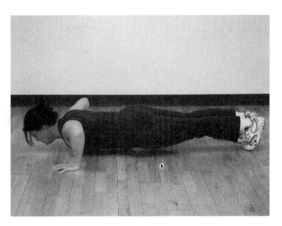

5. Abdominals/Legs.

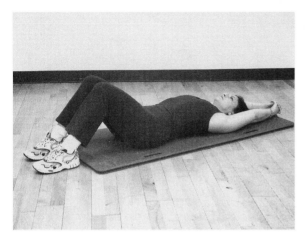

(a) SIT-UPS—75 reps

BEGINNER:

Lie on back with knees bent, feet flat on the floor with heels up against your mat, thumbs clasped with arms extended behind your head. Slowly raise your body all the way up, bringing your chest toward your knees. Exhale while sitting up. Slowly lower body to starting position while inhaling and repeat.

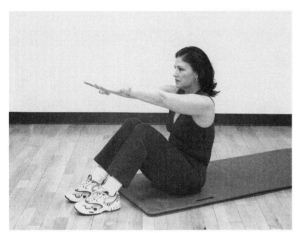

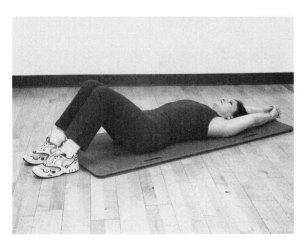

ADVANCED:

Lie on back with knees bent, feet flat on the floor with heels up against your mat, hands on your temples, palms facing in. Slowly raise your body all the way up, bringing your elbows toward your knees. Exhale while sitting up. Slowly lower body to starting position while inhaling and repeat.

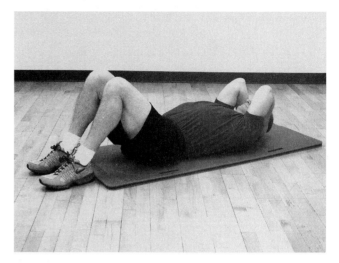

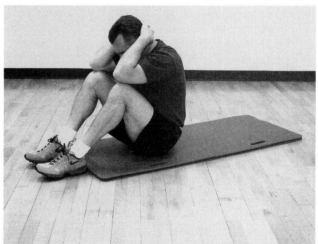

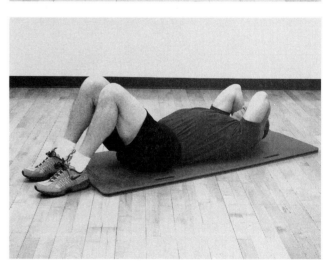

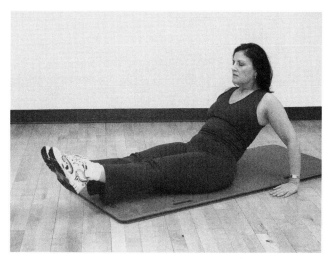

(b) LEG LIFTS—25 reps/25 reps

While sitting back on your buttocks with your hands placed behind you, slightly wider than shoulder width, extend your legs straight in front of you a few inches off the ground. Lift both legs up to 90 degrees. Exhale as you bring your legs upward, making sure that you keep your legs straight throughout entire movement and inhale as you slowly lower legs toward ground. Do not arch back while performing exercise.

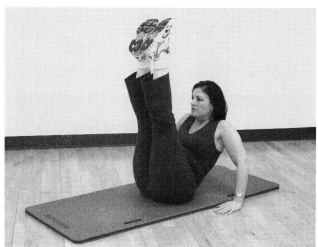

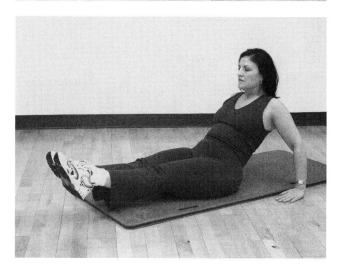

(c) LEG-OUTS—60 reps

Lying on your back, with hands under buttocks, palms down, bring both knees in toward your chest. Slowly straighten legs out with toes pointed and repeat. Inhale while bringing knees toward chest; exhale as you straighten legs. Beginners should straighten legs out at a higher angle. As you get stronger, try to bring legs lower to the ground (about two inches as illustrated) while straightening legs.

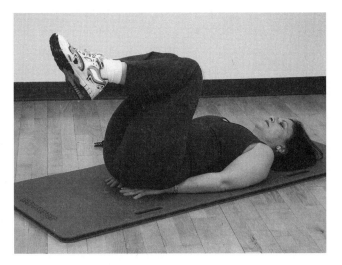

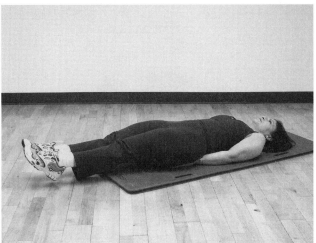

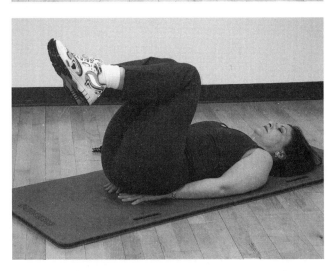

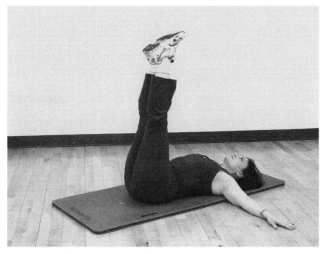

(d) V-SCISSORS (Women only)—50 to 60 reps

Lie on your back, hands at your side or under your buttocks with palms facing down. Raise both legs to 90 degrees. Pressing your back into the floor and with toes pointed and legs straight, slowly open legs as far as possible while exhaling. Bring legs back together, keeping toes pointed and legs straight as you inhale and repeat.

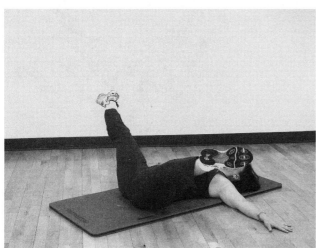

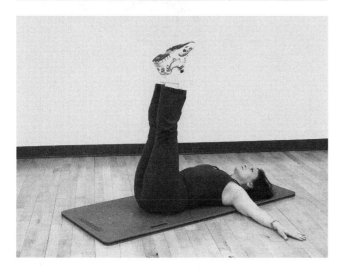

(e) ALTERNATES—75 to 100 reps

Lie on your back with your hands under your buttocks or clasped behind your neck, palms down with legs straight and toes pointed. Raise your right leg to a 90-degree angle, your left leg remaining near the floor. Pressing the small of your back into the floor, lower your right leg as you simultaneously lift your left leg to 90 degrees. Repeat this continuous scissoring motion.

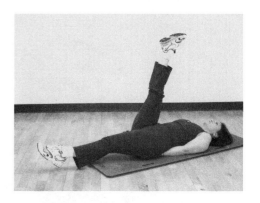

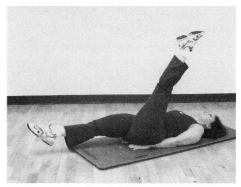

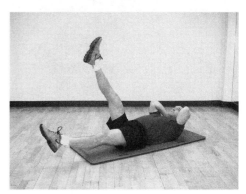

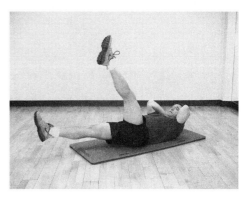

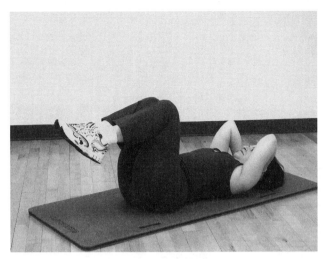

(f) ELBOWS TO KNEES—40 reps

Lying on back, raise knees and feet toward chest in a tucked position. Clasp your hands at the base of your neck. Gently curl your upper body, bringing your elbows toward knees while exhaling. Slowly lower back and shoulders to mat while inhaling and repeat. Keep lower half of your body motionless.

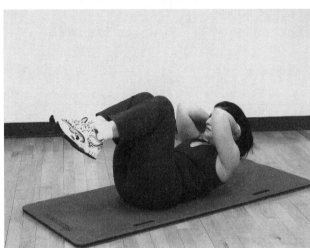

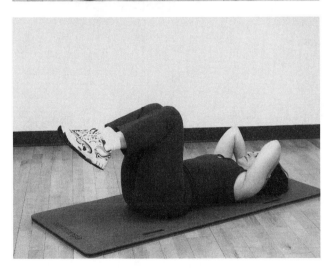

(g) KNEES TO ELBOWS—40 reps

Lying on your back, with hands clasped at the base of your neck, raise head and shoulders off the mat. Raise knees and feet in a tucked position toward elbows, keeping lower back pressed to the floor. Keeping tucked, lower your toes to the ground and repeat. Exhale as you raise knees to elbows; inhale as you lower toes to ground.

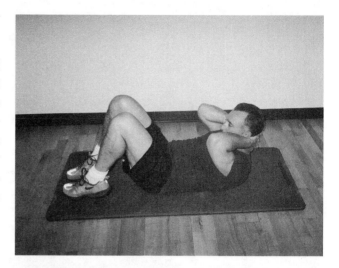

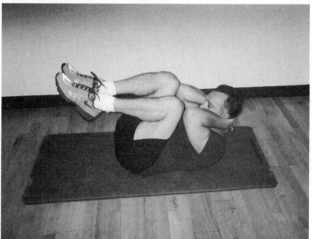

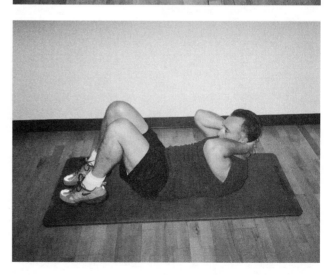

6. Legs/Buttocks.

**Please note: For lower body exercises, you may use either the aerobic toning bar or weighted bar. If you do not want to bulk up, use the aerobic toning bar and just perform more repetitions.

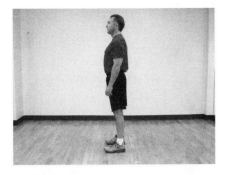

(a) SQUAT THRUSTS—20 to 30 reps

i. Stand with back straight, knees slightly flexed, and feet shoulder width apart.

ii. Bending knees approximately seventy-five degrees into a squat position: (keep thighs parallel with the floor), place palms facedown 8 inches in front of toes and slightly wider than shoulder width.

iii. Exhaling, kick both legs out behind you, landing toes on the floor and legs fully straight and extended.

iv. Thrust back to position ii, then stand up with back straight as you inhale to position i.

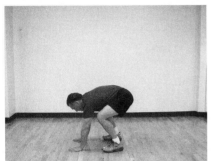

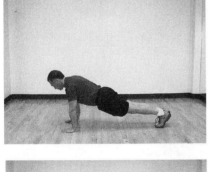

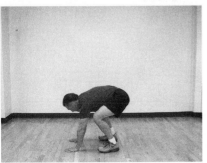

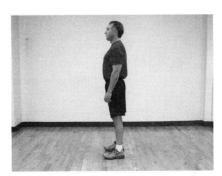

(b) LUNGES (with weighted bar)—20 to 30 reps for each leg

Place either the aerobic toning bar or weighted bar on back of the neck across your shoulders, hands shoulder width apart or more.

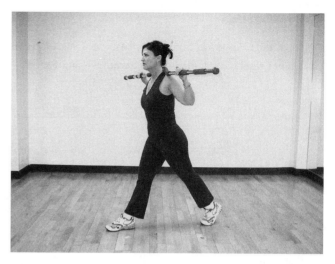

i. Place feet hip width apart and point toes straight ahead and step forward with right leg slightly farther than average stride length, landing foot heel to toe and coming to a complete stop.

ii Keep torso erect; inhale and descend by bending knees and dropping hips straight down, stopping short of left knee touching the ground.

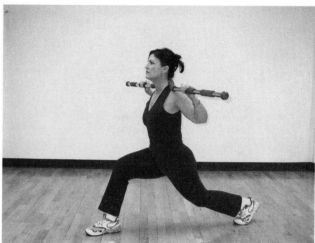

iii. While exhaling, push off right leg and return to starting position with feet hip width apart.

iv. Switch legs and repeat.

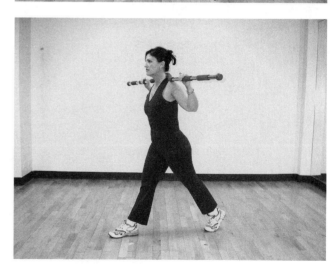

(c) DEAD LIFTS (with aerobic or weighted bar)—40 to 50 reps

Grip either aerobic toning bar or weighted bar with palms facing front of body about shoulder width apart.

i. Hold bar with arms fully extended at front of thighs, elbows at your sides. Feet together or about six inches apart and knees slightly flexed.

ii. Keeping the bar close to the front of your legs, inhale while slowly lowering upper body toward toes as far as possible. Legs should remain slightly bent throughout entire movement.

iii. While exhaling, raise upper body to starting position keeping arms fully extended, back straight and bar close to your body. Squeeze buttocks as your body straightens.

*As flexibility increases, straightening legs (do not lock), stand on a ledge, mat, or step while performing dead lifts will make the exercise more intense by lowering bar below your toes.

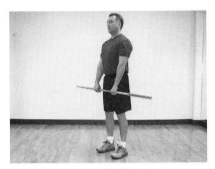 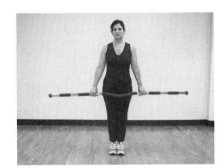

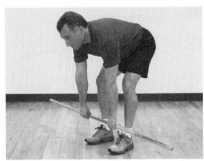 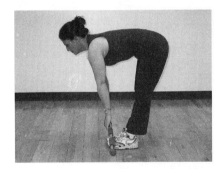

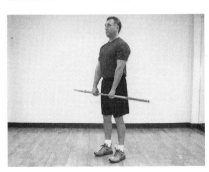 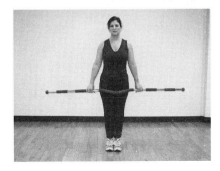

(a) STANDING KNEE TO OPPO-SITE CHEST—50 reps each leg

Rest the aerobic toning bar on your neck across your shoulders, with feet shoulder width apart.

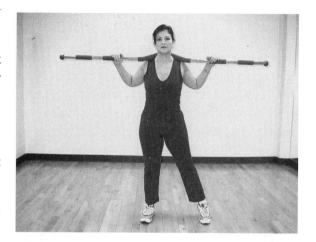

i.   Transfer all weight to your left leg.

ii. Raise right knee up toward your left chest to at least waist-chest level.

iii. Lower right foot to starting position, touching the ground while keeping your weight on your left leg throughout the movement. Switch legs and repeat.

iv. Try to keep aerobic bar straight across back/shoulders while performing exercise.

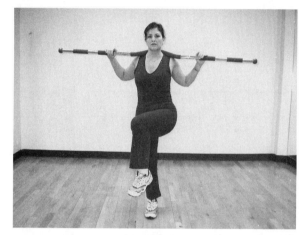

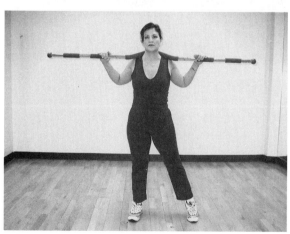

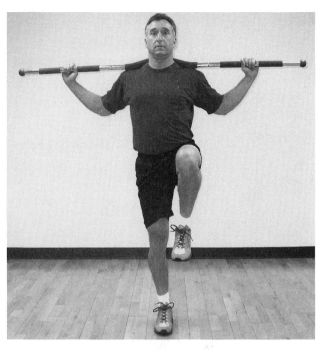

(b) MARCH IN PLACE ON TOES—100 reps

Rest the aerobic toning bar across your shoulders with feet about shoulder width apart and raise up to your toes.

i. Raise left knee straight up to at least waist level toward your chest. Keep back straight and abdominals contracted.

ii. Lower left leg to starting position to toes, making sure that your heels do not touch ground throughout entire movement

iii. Alternate legs through entire exercise.

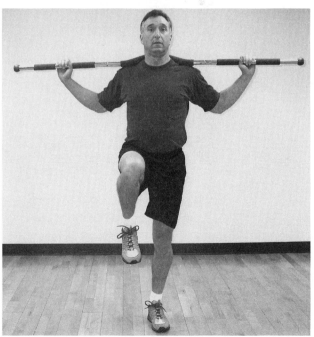

8. Upper Body Exercise.

**Please note: For upper body exercises, you may use either the aerobic toning bar or weighted bar. If you do not want to bulk up, use the aerobic toning bar and just perform more repetitions.

(a) PUSH-OUTS—30 reps
Keep back straight, knees slightly flexed, and feet shoulder width apart.

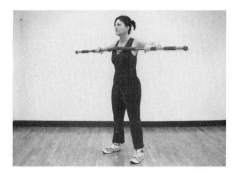

i. Grip bar, palms facing down, just past shoulder width. Raise bar up just above your chest line with elbows up and wrists firm.

ii. Extend arms straight out, holding bar above chest level, and exhale.

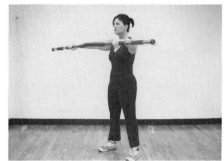

iii. While inhaling, bring bar back to starting position and repeat. Keep lower body aligned and still throughout entire exercise.

iv. Moderate speed throughout entire movement.

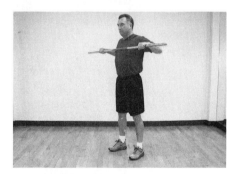

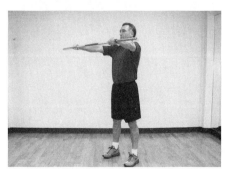

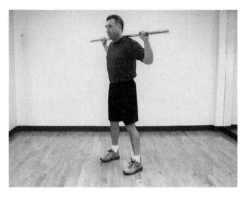

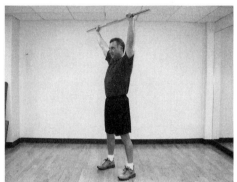

(b) BEHIND THE NECK PRESS—30 reps

Keep back straight, knees slightly flexed, and feet shoulder width apart.

i.   Grip bar just past shoulder width and place behind neck and shoulders.

ii. Fully extend arms and raise bar straight up behind head while exhaling. Bend arms and slowly return bar to behind neck while inhaling and repeat.

iii. Slow speed throughout entire movement.

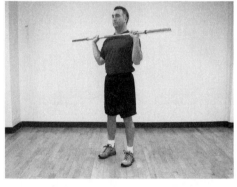

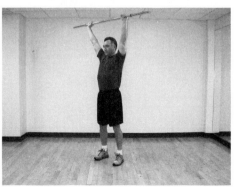

(c) FRONT PRESS—30 reps

Keep back straight, knees flexed, and feet shoulder width apart.

i.   Grip bar just past shoulder width and rest bar across top of chest.

ii. Fully extend arms upward and raise bar straight up while exhaling. Bend arms and slowly return bar to top of chest while inhaling and repeat.

iii. Moderate speed throughout entire movement.

(d) WIDE UPRIGHT ROWS—30 reps

Keep back straight, knees slightly flexed, and feet shoulder width apart.

i. Grip bar, palms facing down, hands shoulder width apart. Hold bar with arms fully extended at front of thighs.

ii. Slowly raise bar up to chin, keeping elbows at or above bar level while exhaling. Return to starting position while inhaling and repeat.

iii. Moderate speed throughout entire movement.

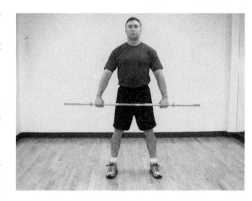

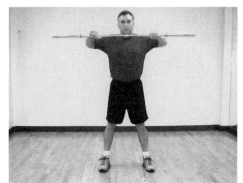

(e) NARROW UPRIGHT ROWS—30 reps

Keep back straight, knees slightly flexed, and feet shoulder width apart.

i. Grip bar, palms facing down, hands six to eight inches apart. Hold bar with arms fully extended at front of thighs.

ii. Slowly raise bar to chin, keeping elbows at or above bar level while exhaling. Return to starting position while inhaling and repeat.

iii. Moderate speed throughout entire movement.

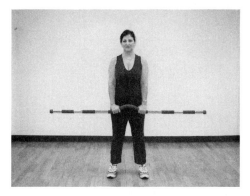

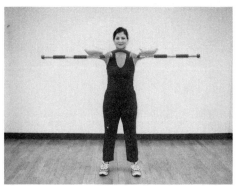

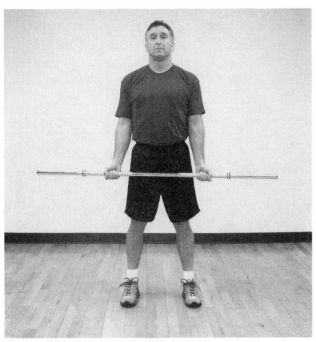

(f) CURLS—30 reps

Keep back straight, knees flexed, and feet shoulder width apart.

i. Grip bar, palms facing up and shoulder width apart. Hold bar with arms fully extended at front of thighs.

ii. Keeping elbows stationary and wrists firm, curl bar up to chest while exhaling. Slowly extend arms and return bar to start position while inhaling and repeat.

iii. Moderate speed throughout entire movement.

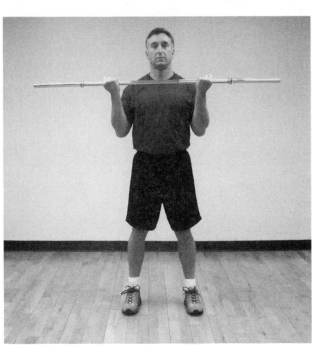

(g) KICK-BACKS—30 reps

Keep back straight, knees slightly flexed, and feet shoulder width apart.

i. Grip bar with arms fully extended at buttocks, palms facing outward about shoulder width apart.

ii. Keeping elbows stationary and wrists firm, raise bar away from your buttocks as far as possible while exhaling. Keeping arms straight, lower bar to buttocks while inhaling and repeat.

iii. Moderate speed throughout entire movement.

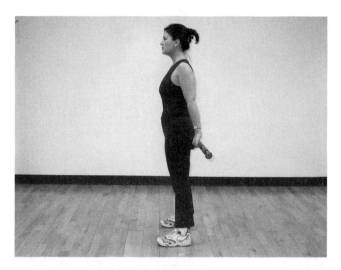

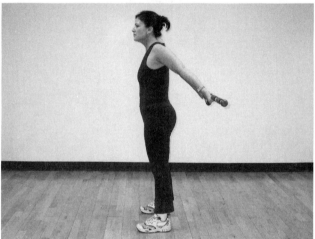

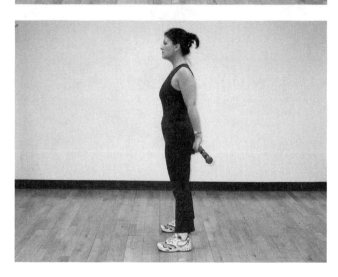

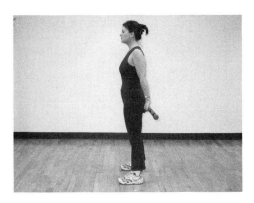

(h) ADVANCED KICK-BACKS—20 reps

Keep back straight, knees slightly flexed, and feet shoulder width apart.

i. Grip bar with arms fully extended at buttocks, palms facing outward about shoulder width apart.

ii. Keeping wrists firm, bend arms and raise bar away from your buttocks as far as possible while exhaling. Keeping arms straight, lower bar to buttocks while inhaling and repeat.

iii. Moderate speed throughout entire movement.

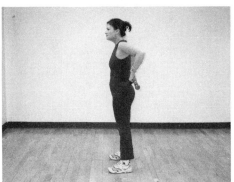

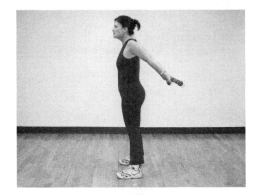

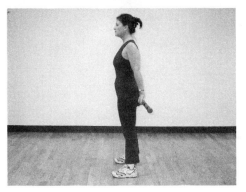

9. Legs/Buttocks.

(a) SQUAT THRUSTS—20 reps

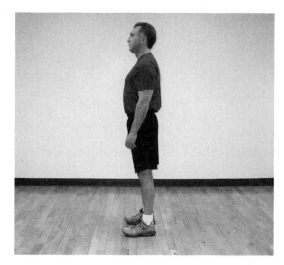

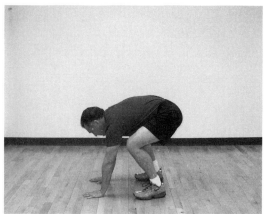

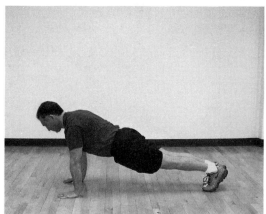

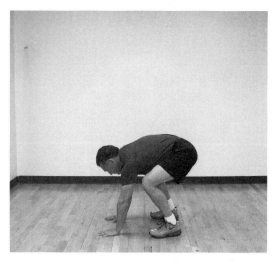

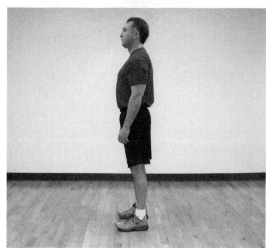

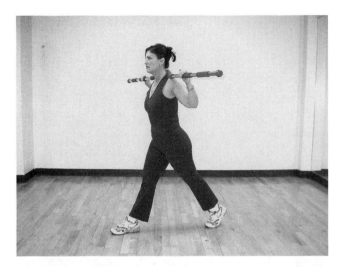

(b) LUNGES—20 reps

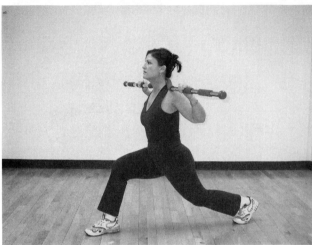

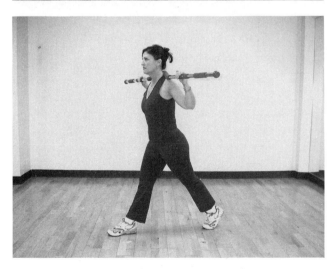

(c) DEAD LIFTS—40 reps

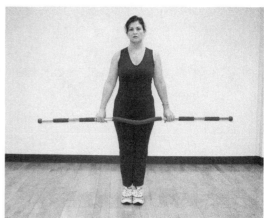

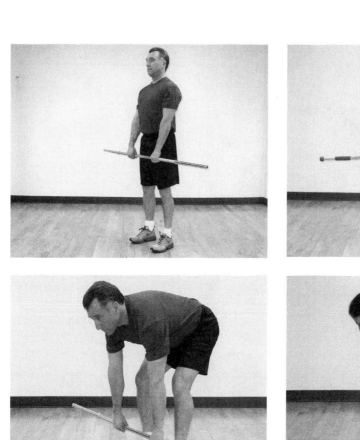

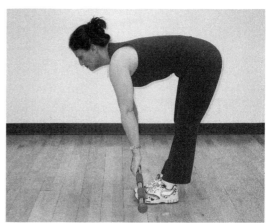

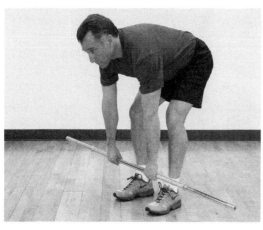

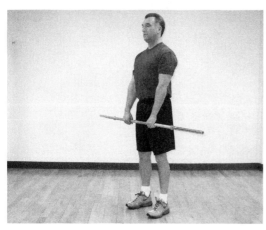

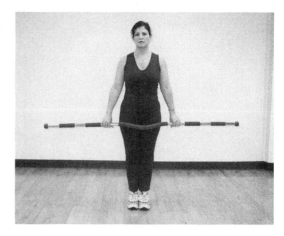

10. Fat Burner—7 minutes of jumping rope or 3 minutes of marching in place on toes, then 4 minutes of favorite aerobic piece of equipment of your choice, vigorously!

JUMPING ROPE–7 minutes

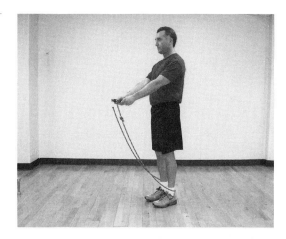

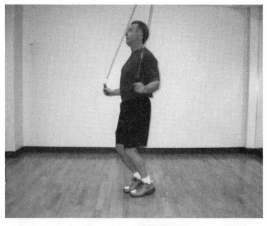

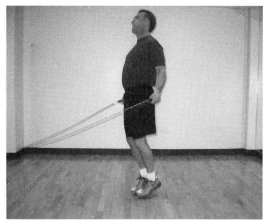

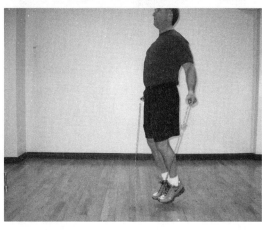

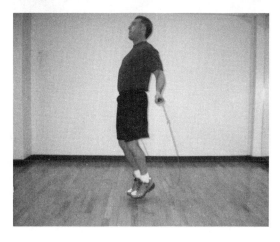

OR MARCHING IN PLACE ON TOES—3 MINUTES

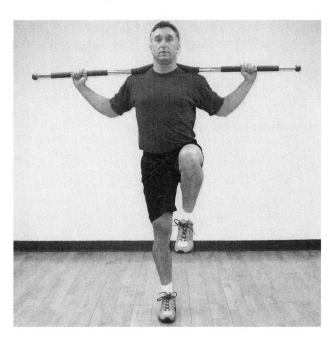

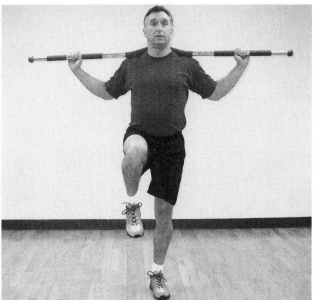

4 MINUTES OF AEROBIC EXERCISE

11. Cooldown—3 minutes of walking or biking leisurely.

Workout #2—See page 222 for additional Off Day Routine prescription.

Additional Exercises

UPPER BODY

BENT OVER ROWS

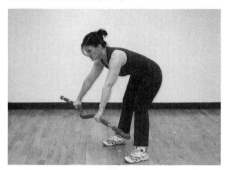

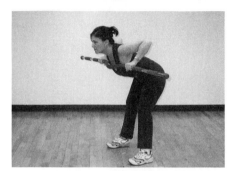

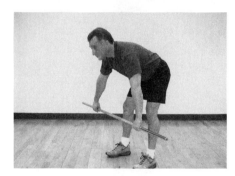

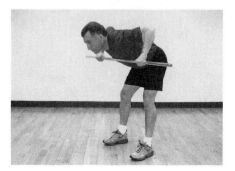

CHAIR DIPS

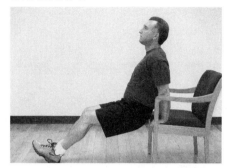

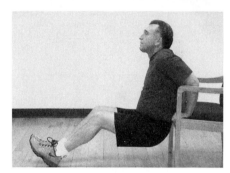

TWISTER SIT-UPS

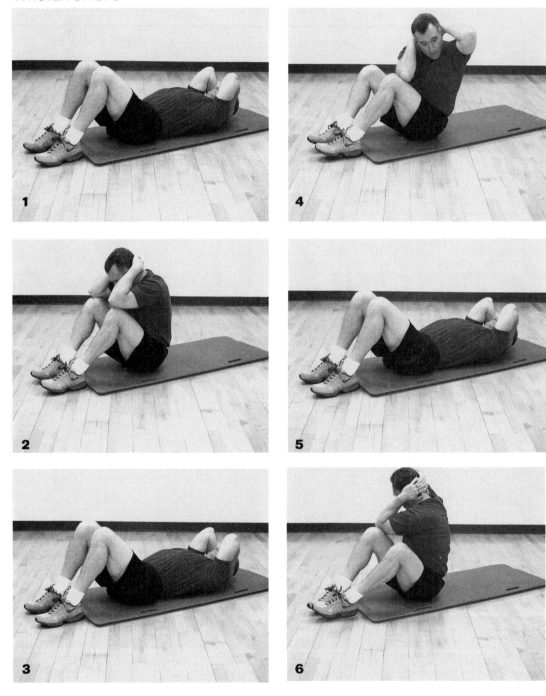

SIDE LEG LIFTS

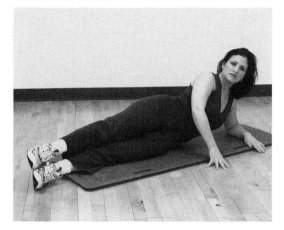

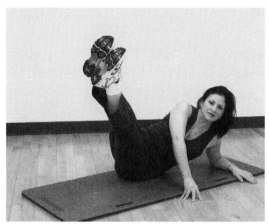

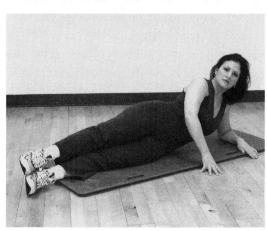

ANGLED LEG-OUTS

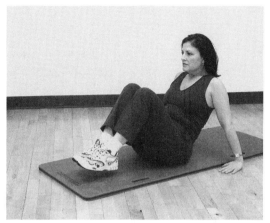

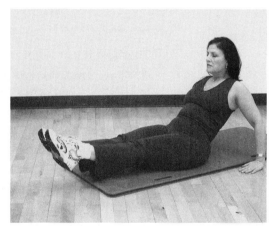

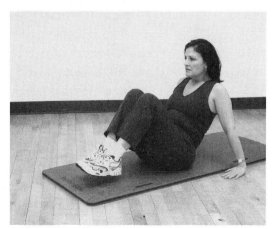

CHAPTER NINE

Conclusion and Height/Weight Chart

Conclusion

The most important thing to keep in mind when trying to lose weight is choosing the right approach that you can be consistent with over the long haul. Then, after you have chosen the path that plays to your strengths, it is equally important to not deviate from the recipe of success that I've outlined for you. Most people are not aware that they need to accept the fact that weight loss and weight management is something that they need to focus on probably for the rest of their lives. The *key* is to counterpunch when you have bad eating days by performing 30–45 minutes of aerobic exercise to rid your body of those extra calories you've consumed to get back to the scale weight you were before you got off track. Remember, you can only gain weight if you take in and consume more calories than you burn off through your activities and exercise routine. And everyone, despite how disciplined you may think you are, will have days when you overeat and/or overdrink or days when you just don't feel like moving—it's normal. That's why it is so important to have a few activities sprinkled into your lifestyle, because the more fit you are, the more active you will be. If you are feeling too tired or just don't feel like working out, at least you did something active that particular day, and if you do gain weight, it may just be a pound versus 2–3 pounds by not moving, coupled with a poor-eating day.

Another thing I've noticed is that we tend to eat much healthier on the days that we workout. The reason that we are more conscious about our dietary habits on days when we exercise is because we have done something positive for our bodies and minds that particular day, so we don't want to sabotage ourselves. Additionally, movement and sweating helps fight that lethargic feeling we sometimes feel as well as getting us out of a funky or depressed mood. That's why whenever I feel down or lazy, I just start moving, and within a half-hour or so, I am in such a better state of mind. Also, the more you move and/or exercise, the less time and fewer opportunities you have for eating.

By being very active and exercising with a lot of frequency, you can also look at food and drink as a reward system. Whatever your motivation is to lose weight or approach you take to shed pounds, it doesn't matter how you do it, as long as it is done in a healthy manner and something that you can mimic on a day-in-and-day-out basis.

So, the next time you see, read, or hear an advertisement on how easy it is to lose weight by just exercising a few minutes a day and/or by taking a magical pill or potion, stop and think for a moment. Think logically; if it were so easy and effective to lose weight, then there would be no overweight and out-of-shape people, including you.

The main reason why so few people exercise with regularity is because they have never followed the recipe and format that's needed to gain the benefits from fitness. Review chapter 3 and you'll have a better understanding of what I mean. It is imperative that you follow the four phases of a workout and exercise in a manner that improves all five components of fitness each and every time you exercise, so that you're guaranteed to feel great and realize all the profits from your hard work and efforts. As you get closer and draw nearer toward your weight-loss goals, keep in mind that you are building lifelong eating and exercise habits that will remain with you for many years to come. When and if you do happen to get "off track" with either your eating or fitness, don't despair, don't pity yourself, or get disappointed with your results. Instead, put it behind you and focus on what you need to do to get back in the game by eating sensibly and exercising regularly. Also, if you hit a "plateau" during anytime with your weight-loss goals, it's most likely because you are not exercising with enough intensity and/or you need to make adjustments with your diet in order to keep creating that deficit of calories—which is the *only* way to lose and keep weight off, whether it's 1, 10, or 50 pounds.

And remember, the short cut, my friend, is learning how to eat sensibly and exercise consistently and properly. By doing so, you will see fast results—and results that will help you achieve a lifetime of possessing a fit, toned, and healthy body!

If you need further assistance with your weight-loss objectives or have a question regarding your diet and/or exercise regimen, e-mail us at *info@exude.com* or log onto our Web site at *www.exude.com* to order any fitness-related tools needed to help you escape your weight. You may also write us at:

Attn: Program Director
EXUDE Fitness
16 East 52nd Street, 3rd Floor
New York, N.Y. 10022
1-800-24-EXUDE or 212-644-9559

Height/Weight Chart

I've created and put together for you a new Height/Weight Chart for both men and women based on your frame: small, medium, or large. This is based upon my experience of working with over 20,000 clients over the years. This is what I feel is a realistic weight for each height based on the size of your frame. The smaller your frame, the less you should weigh, and you should strive toward that number. Conversely, the larger-framed you are, the more weight you can carry. Also, these weight ranges are based on the fact that you are fit and possess a healthy body fat percentage: Men: 8–17 percent and women: 12–22 percent.

Men		
Height–Inches	Maximum Weight–Lbs. (Small–Medium Frame)	Maximum Weight–Lbs. (Large Frame)
5'2"	118	130
5'3"	121	135
5'4"	124	140
5'5"	127	145
5'6"	131	150
5'7"	135	160
5'8"	139	170
5'9"	150	180
5'10"	155	190
5'11"	160	200
6'0"	165	205
6'1"	170	210
6'2"	175	215
6'3"	185	225
6'4"	195	235
6'5"	205	245

Women		
Height–Inches	Maximum Weight–Lbs. (Small–Medium Frame)	Maximum Weight–Lbs. (Large Frame)
4'9"	96	111
4'10"	99	114
4'11"	102	117
5'0"	105	120
5'1"	108	123
5'2"	111	126
5'3"	114	129
5'4"	118	133
5'5"	122	137
5'6"	126	142
5'7"	128	144
5'8"	132	148
5'9"	135	155
5'10"	140	160
5'11"	145	165
6'0"	150	170

CHAPTER TEN

Testimonials and Pictures

Carolyn Makuen—11–30 Weight Loss

One day in September 2002, I went to a seminar (paid for by my employer) about "Emotional Discipline and Self-Control." The class was taught by a man about my age who had a fascinating personal/career history in motivational speaking and coaching as well as "extreme sports," such as ultratriathlons in extreme climates. It was the first seminar in which I never experienced any sleepiness; I was riveted by the man's energy and anecdotes. He asked the whole class, "What's the secret to weight loss and fitness?" and everyone replied in unison, "Eat right and exercise." He replied, "And yet every bookstore and library is crammed full of books on gimmicky diets and fitness regimens, and television constantly runs infomercials for Ab Busters." What a powerful commentary this was on the futility of human existence! And there I sat, a naturally slender person who has battled my whole life against a bulging abdomen from an intestinal disease (celiac disease or sprue). My wrists are 5.5 inches around, but I'm wearing a size 14. Something was out of whack given my habits of healthy eating and regular exercise, including power-walks and ab work.

Five days later, I waited an hour and a quarter in a New York City doctor's office where the reading material was of very little interest to me. In an old *New York* magazine, there was a small blurb about Dr. Ed Jackowski's exercise theories, his gym in New York City, and the books he has written on the subject. Something clicked in my brain ("Eat right and exercise," from the seminar the week before, and the article's quotations from women whose butts got bigger after workouts on steppers).

After being so late at the doctor that night, I had a gap of time until the next train (the train schedule runs the commuter's life in New York City), and I popped into a bookstore. The rest, as they say, is history. I read the books *Escape Your Shape* and *Hold It! You're Exercising Wrong!* that night. Some of the most appealing concepts were Edward's recognition that one needed an exercise regimen that was practical and consistent and that there was no need for a lot of elaborate equipment because "these are exercises you learned in third grade gym class." I wanted to get down on the floor that night and start my program! The next day I made an appointment for a fitness assessment at the Exude facility, which I found was a mere four blocks from my New York City office, with the president, Lee Ross.

Edward, Lee, and the staff gave me intense personal attention during my introductory fitness assessment. I had never had one-on-one attention in front of a mirror while exercising (even in gym class there were always thirty other kids). It was easy to see that paying an Exude trainer for more of this attention on a regular basis would be worthwhile. The Polaroids and measurements were taken, and I bought an exercise bike for my house within days so that I could keep up with the homework I was prescribed by Exude. I knew I could make my newfound exercise routine a habit by creating a little gym in my basement. I made sure I could watch my favorite television shows (taped) while I worked out. This made the time investment dual-purpose and coincided well with the new fall TV season.

After four weeks of my new Exude exercise regimen, I had lost "seven inches from my bad places" (as I told family and friends). Everyone gave me the "muscle weighs more than fat" adage when I complained of having lost no weight in those four weeks. Coincidentally, at the same time on October 31, 2002, an old friend began pestering me to try a new diet. I whined about every tenet of her diet, to the extent that my friend said, "Get the book, just try it, and if you don't lose weight by Thanksgiving, I'll give you the money back you spent on the book." I agreed, just to get her off my back! It was combining the proper exercise and diet that allowed me to shed the pounds as well as more inches. Needless to say, the $20 I spent for the book was a wise investment. I owe my friend some flowers.

My new diet regimen encouraged me to drop the highly glycemic carbs to which I was addicted (white basmati rice, potatoes, and corn in the form of tortillas). I can still eat lots of delicious carbs as long as they're whole grain and not combined with fats/proteins. I continued with the Exude workouts and have shed 12 pounds in ten weeks. I now know I will not "die a size 14." I cannot wait until my fortieth birthday when I'll be happy, for the first time in my life, with my body. I highly recommend the Escape Your Weight regimen to all.

NAME: Carolyn Makuen

DATE: January 9, 2003

AGE: 39

TOTAL INCHES LOST: 20.75

TOTAL WEIGHT LOST: 22.50 pounds

TIME IT TOOK TO LOSE THE WEIGHT: 10–15 weeks

PRIOR EXERCISE REGIMEN: Vigorous walk (2 miles in 28 minutes) 2–3 times per week, plus 15 minutes of abs 3 times per week, plus yoga once per week. Prior goal was to enjoy being outdoors and keep up with my family legacy of being fast walkers. Always hoped to slim down but the exercise seemed to do nothing in that vein. One year of abs work seemed pointless.

CURRENT EXERCISE REGIMEN: Customized workouts for my needs, once per week with an Exude trainer, 3–5 additional home workouts, plus yoga once per week.

PRIOR EATING HABITS: Gluten-free (no wheat/rye/oats/barley) omnivore. Did not diet, but was always a very healthy eater, avoiding processed foods and added sugars. A big fan of high starches like rice, potatoes, and corn.

CURRENT EATING HABITS: The main changes in my diet include no combining carbs with proteins/fats, fruit eaten by itself only, and no "funky foods" (none of the rice, potatoes, or corn to which I was "addicted"). This worked well for me and my digestion process, especially given my intestinal disease (celiac disease).

THE MAIN FACTOR THAT HELPED CAROLYN TO ESCAPE HER WEIGHT: My consistent Exude workouts, motivation and reinforcement from Exude staff, and dieting (which my body seemed to need as a big "shock" or change to lifelong eating habits).

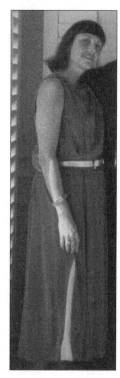
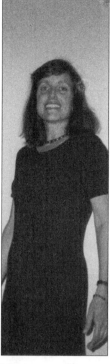

Carolyn Makuen

Camille Sinclair—60-Plus Weight Loss

There are no memories of my childhood and adolescent years where I have not been overweight/obese. I can comprise a list of the ill effects that being overweight has had on my self esteem; however, my initial reasons for losing weight were health-related. I could neither run without my knees, ankles, and lower back being sore, nor could I run up a flight of stairs without wheezing. One winter, after having several weather-and-weight-related asthma attacks in a month, my physician seriously advised me to begin a diet and exercise routine to lose weight and increase my fitness level.

As per my doctor's warnings, I substituted high-fat foods for lower-fat and healthier choices. I also began exercise workouts at home. Within a few months, I lost some weight but quickly plateaued. After much research, it became clear that Exude Fitness was the best place for me. Dr. Jackowski impressed me with his knowledge of various body compositions and how best to tailor an exercise routine accordingly. The Exude methodology was just what the doctor ordered (no pun intended)!!

Not only did a lot of additional pounds peel off with my new diet and Exude workout routines, but my fitness level also went through the roof! Now I can effortlessly dodge up a flight of stairs, jump rope for 15–20 minutes, and out run many of my slimmer (but not necessarily fitter) friends. I feel so much healthier and look forward to reaching my long-term goal weight with Exude. Thank you!!

NAME: Camille Sinclair

DATE: January 24, 2003

AGE: 23

TOTAL INCHES LOST: n/a

TOTAL WEIGHT LOST: 77 pounds

TIME IT TOOK TO LOSE THE WEIGHT: Two years

PRIOR EXERCISE REGIMEN: Elliptical, step machine, and treadmill routines 1–2 times per week for 30–45 minutes.

CURRENT EXERCISE REGIMEN: Personalized Exude workout, which incorporates warm-up, stretch, workload, and cooldown routines, 4 days a week on my own.

EATING HABITS PRIOR TO WEIGHT LOSS: High-fat, sugar, and carbohydrate meals (i.e., deep-fried chicken, French fries, lasagna, whole milk, et cetera).

CURRENT EATING HABITS: Baked, broiled, and roasted lean protein; reduced-fat dairy; high-fiber carbohydrates, fruits, vegetables, et cetera.

THE MAIN FACTOR THAT HELPED CAMILLE ESCAPE HER WEIGHT: Nutritional counseling as well as the customized Exude workouts were integral factors to my weight loss. The Exude routines have also toned my problem areas, thereby eliminating loose skin that frequently accompanies major weight loss.

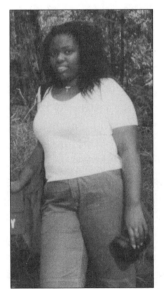 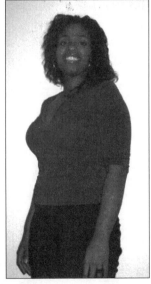

Camille Sinclair

Pamala McCormick-Steward—10 and Under Weight Loss

When I was about ten years old, I found that I was becoming bigger and curvier than my own mother, and that didn't seem right. She said she wished she had my hips, but I would have gladly exchanged my hips for hers. Standing 5' 7" and 140 pounds besides my mother's petite 102-pound frame, I felt like a monstrosity.

As an only child, and an introvert at heart in a single-and-often-absent-parent household, I spent most of my time alone and terribly lonely. Food gratified me. While watching television reruns and doing homework, I could easily wolf down bowl after bowl of Honey Nut Cheerios, the remaining leftovers of a Sara Lee apple pie, 3–5 peanut-butter-and-jelly sandwiches, or several slices of buttered toast. I could never eat just one of any of my favorite foods or I'd feel a powerful sense of deprivation and obsess about it until I could no longer resist eating it in its entirety.

At junior high school, most of us girls compared our weights and the expanse of our thighs on the seat of chairs. Mine seemed one of the highest. I desired to be skinny, skinnier than my mother.

I studied a variety of diet-related books and magazines and often went for days on end subsisting only on tea. When I absolutely couldn't resist my mother's spaghetti and meat sauce or some other food, I ate my fill of it and then vomited it up. Although I cleaned up as best as I could, my mother caught on and asked me if I was throwing up. "Oh no," I lied, "Not me." I was ashamed.

I fasted and dieted until I didn't have any fat to keep me warm anymore. My collarbone jutted out from my chest, and my pants swam around my waist. At around age sixteen, close friends chided me that I was too small and pushed plates of southern home cooking in my face. I was moved that they cared and, as a thank you, began to eat in large portions again.

My weight stayed in the 116–120 range until my first pregnancy. The obstetrician advised me to gain weight, and I happily obliged, eating to my heart's desire. By the time I entered the hospital to give birth, I tipped the scales at around 183 pounds. Home from the hospital two days later, and horribly swollen and misshapen, I desperately began to exercise, much to my family's horror. "You're going to hurt yourself," they warned. I appreciated their concern, but they couldn't possibly understand how heavy and grotesque I felt. A woman wasn't supposed to weigh as much as a man. I did step aerobics over an hour a day and ate as little as possible. On a "good" day, I ate nothing. I was proud of myself when I reported to work two months later 44 pounds lighter and still losing.

This cycle continued to a lesser and lesser extent after each of my next two pregnancies. I no longer had the energy and control to obsess about my weight. Furthermore, singer Karen Carpenter's death drove home the fact that what I had been doing to my body could kill me.

My weight eventually stabilized around 126 pounds—6 pounds over my personal weight preference. No big deal. Then over a seven-month period, I was shrouded by a profound depression precipitated by a dispute with my father-in-law. My conscientiousness about my weight went to hell, and I began to gain weight. My in-laws and I co-own our home, and every day I struggled with the decision of whether to leave or stay with my husband and three girls. My father-in-law and I were not talking, and I found coming home to face-off with the tension and strife close to intolerable. Desperate for some psychological relief, I sought help and was treated with therapy and medication, which helped me to emerge out of the depression in a couple of months with newfound coping skills, but 17 pounds heavier.

When the Body Challenge competition was announced at my company, there was no question that I was going to participate. I love to follow a positive course of action and friendly competition. I cobbled together a team and sent off application forms to Human Resources. Dr. Edward Jackowski, CEO of Exude Fitness, and Lee Ross, president of Exude Fitness, one of the largest motivational one-on-one fitness companies in the country oversaw the Body Challenge program, along with their team of professionals. I studied the Exude.com Web site, read Edward's books, and listened to the audiotapes. Exude's philosophy and support caused me to reframe what I thought about my body and weight loss. I never cared about the idea of getting fit before—fitness was for athletes. When I read about the five components of fitness: cardiovascular health, muscle strength, muscle endurance, flexibility, and lean muscle to fat ratio, the idea of becoming fit became accessible, and I wanted that for myself. I knew from experience what "skinny fat" was like, and I didn't want to lose a lot of weight and flap in the wind.

After embarking on this newfound workout regimen specifically designed to meet my specific needs, I noticed results immediately. I lost pounds *and* inches. After a few weeks, my body seemed to recall some of the cardiovascular progress I had made back when I was doing step aerobics. My stomach tightened in a way I have never seen since having children. My energy level increased. I looked forward to exercising, not because I liked it (because I don't), but to facilitate my body's capacity to overcome resistance of all types and better tolerate day-to-day stresses. At one point, my weight plateaued for over a month. If this had been a decade ago, I would have bullishly starved to make the scale move. But after venting my frustrations with Lee Ross, I received the encouragement and, more important, the guidance I needed to remedy the plateau by actually eating more and providing the extra calories my body needed to burn fat.

Now I have a new respect for my body. I delight in its shape and am learning how to flatter it with makeup and certain clothing styles. I'm never going to forsake my precious health again with obsessive dieting over exercising and abusive habits. There are no guarantees, but I'm determined to continue to do all that I can to contribute to my having a long, healthy, and productive life.

NAME: Pamala McCormick-Steward

DATE: August 28, 2003

AGE: 33

TOTAL INCHES LOST: 17

TOTAL WEIGHT LOST: 18 pounds

TIME IT TOOK TO LOSE THE WEIGHT: 70 days

PRIOR EXERCISE REGIMEN: Jane Fonda's 45-minute Step Aerobic Workout routine on an inconsistent basis, mostly after the births of my three daughters.

CURRENT EXERCISE REGIMEN: My workout is an intense full-body routine and incorporates upper- and lower-body work as well as abdominals and cardio in the beginning and end. I usually try to exercise 5–6 days per week, including full-body calisthenics, a two-mile walk 2–3 times per week during the workday, and then add in the jump rope 3 other days per week when I am at home. I had a metabolic test taken so that I could establish an accurate daily-caloric range that would allow me to lose weight. I adhered to this calorie budget, and I slowly dropped those extra pounds without feeling hungry or having to stifle cravings.

PRIOR EATING HABITS: During the work week, I would not have time to eat a lot, so I stuck to pita sandwiches, pasta dishes, and salads. On the weekends, I ate whatever I wanted without being too concerned about calories, southern-style buttermilk biscuits, McDonald's extra-value meals, Chili's boneless buffalo wings and nachos, and Red Lobster's cheddar cheese biscuits and fried seafood.

CURRENT EATING HABITS: Since I am exercising consistently, I don't deprive myself of my favorite foods; I just make sure to stick to my daily-calorie limit. That being said, I'm less likely to eat a Big Mac and fries now, as it would blow away my budget for the whole day! To maintain progress, I prefer not to eat something I don't know the nutritional information of, so I weigh and calculate almost everything. I like prepacked meals, since it eliminates the guesswork. Usually, I enjoy a low-carb, protein-packed Atkins bar, whole wheat cereal, or skillet potatoes made with Pam cooking spray for breakfast. Lunch is a Lean Cuisine entrée or a green salad. Dinner is a turkey or garden burger, a Lean Cuisine entrée, or even a potpie. I snack on nuts, popcorn, and prepackaged low-carb snacks. When I go over my calorie budget, I either exercise more and/or eat less the following day. I also take a calcium supplement and a multivitamin.

THE MAIN FACTOR THAT HELPED PAMALA TO ESCAPE HER WEIGHT: Understanding my individual exercise and calorie requirements as they related to my specific needs and metabolism and following my prescribed Exude exercise program 4–6 days per week. I have motivated myself to work out completely on my own!

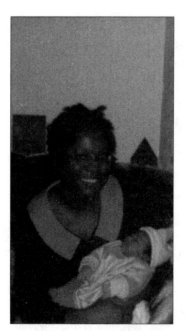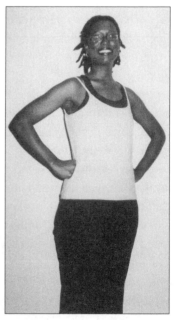

Pamala McCormick-Steward

Lori Isola-Montuori—10 and Under Weight Loss

Yes, I enjoy exercising. I joined a gym at age thirty-six and began a consistent five-days-a-week schedule. I wanted to lose 20 pounds and was hooked when the weight started coming off. I would do 60 minutes of cardio using a bike, treadmill, or combination, followed by a half hour to an hour of weight training. Each trip to the gym left me feeling strong and powerful. I trained hard and was challenged by the heavy weights I could lift. I put on muscle easily and liked how it made me feel. I didn't even really have to change my diet to see results.

Since I knew this routine had worked, I stuck with it, even when, years later, I started gaining weight back. I didn't understand why all the gym time wasn't working anymore. I tried some classes—spinning, yoga, and sculpt. I thought if I just varied what I did, I could relose the 20 pounds I gained. It was extremely frustrating, but I kept with it. That was when Dr. Edward Jackowski approached me at my gym. I had just come off the seated chest-press machine (30 pounds on each side) when he introduced himself and told me about a Web site he wanted me to check out—exude.com. He had seen me in the gym on several occasions doing the wrong types of exercise and thought I would benefit from the methods outlined on the site. He suggested that for my goals I should not be lifting heavy weights, because I was only making my body bigger. I agreed that my body did not have the slim shape I was striving for, so something needed to change.

To say I was intrigued would be an understatement. I checked out exude.com and found the descriptions for my needs and found that I was doing all the things that Edward said I shouldn't be doing to get in shape. I had to learn more and called to make an appointment with Lee, the Exude Fitness president, the next day.

The workouts that Lee created for me were completely different than how I was exercising and very different than any type of exercise I had done in the past. I signed up for a number of sessions and began working with my assigned Exude trainer, Robert. I was highly motivated, challenged, and happy to have a new focus and plan of attack. I couldn't wait until the month was over to be able to measure my results. Now, I've retired my weight gloves and always show up to the gym with my jump rope. I think my fellow gym "regulars" are surprised to see my new fitness routine but are starting to notice a significant change in my body and shape.

I knew the Exude program was working when my clothes started to fit better. I lost 7.5 inches and 4 pounds in the first 5 weeks. I'm extremely pleased with these results and very happy that Edward approached me in the gym. I do miss the power of heavy-weight lifting, but I realize that it's not the way for me to get lean. I enjoy jumping rope and look forward to the personal attention I get at the Exude Fitness facility. You feel like a celebrity being trained for a movie role when you are there. It's great to have a proven fitness plan that provides results as long as you are willing to put in the effort. Since that's never been a problem for me, I look forward to continued success with the Exude team . . . more pound- and inch-loss and some fun along the way.

NAME: Lori Isola-Montuori

DATE: September 8, 2003

AGE: 43

TOTAL INCHES LOST: 7.5

TOTAL WEIGHT LOST: 4 pounds

TIME IT TOOK TO LOSE THE WEIGHT: 5 weeks

PRIOR EXERCISE REGIMEN: An hour of cardio on combination of bike, treadmill, and elliptical machine and a half hour of heavy weights 5 times a week. Would substitute a spin class once a week. I own a Lifecycle bike at home, plus hand weights, an easy-curl bar, yoga ball, and dynabands. I tried to vary my workouts. Lunges and squats for my legs, bar and weight routines for upper body. Exercise gave me more energy, better sleep, and feelings of accomplishment. Felt my efforts weren't showing for the amount of time spent.

CURRENT EXERCISE REGIMEN: I began working out with an Exude trainer 2 times a week who focused on slimming down my overly developed assets by using light weights and more repetitions for my entire body. On my own, I followed the Exude off-day prescription 3 times a week, which included more cardio and light weights with a lot of repetitions and jumping rope.

PRIOR EATING HABITS: Generally healthy, lots of fruits and vegetables. Breakfast is cereal, yogurt, and fruit or some ricotta cheese on toast. Lunch is salads, tuna, egg and turkey sandwiches. Dinner is chicken, fish, and occasionally red meat. I eat a piece of fruit mid-morning and at around 4 PM. Late-night snacking has been difficult to control, often munching on what's in the cupboard: oatmeal, popcorn, peanut butter, cheese, and sorbet.

CURRENT EATING HABITS: Not much different, except trying to reduce pastas and other carbohydrates. Reduce portion sizes and late-night picking.

Redirection of my fitness regimen, strong motivation, positive reinforcement from the Exude staff, and Edward's influence and guidance.

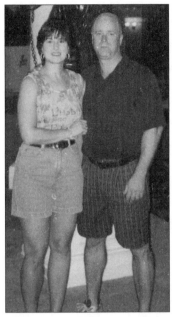 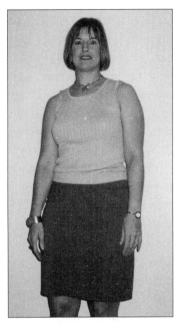

Lori Isola-Montuori

Heather Gallagher—10 and Under Weight Loss

Being an overweight child was always difficult. It was very hard to find the willpower to stick with a diet or exercise program long enough to see any results occur. I would eat as much of anything and everything that I wanted and then get upset because I could never lose weight. The extra weight held me back from participating in activities and doing things that I wanted to do because I felt that people were looking and commenting on the way I looked. Once college came and I realized that being overweight was holding me back from enjoying the best years of my life, I decided that I had had enough! I knew I needed to begin exercising and losing the weight properly once and for all.

For years I had trained with numerous personal trainers, spending up to two hours a day at the gym. Initially, the workouts helped get rid of some excess weight, but I still felt frustrated with my body and dieting left me feeling unsatisfied. I still had 15–20 pounds that I needed to lose. The problem was that the weight lifting program was bulking me up, so the results were not as obvious or what I wanted. Once I stopped seeing the results, my dedication and motivation dissipated, and I felt the same cycle of losing and gaining weight and inches coming back again. It was all too familiar and disappointing.

Then one day I saw an article in a newspaper about Exude Fitness that caught my interest, and I figured that it couldn't hurt to look further into their methodology. I immediately called up and scheduled an appointment for my mom and me to go into New York City and do a fitness assessment. We figured that the program director may be able to show us a few different exercises to add to the ones we already were doing and that would be the end of it. But after the consultation, we were hooked. We walked out feeling that after one hour we were actually accomplishing exactly what we needed to do. When I used to work out at the gym on my previous program, my intensity level peaked only at certain times during the workout. The difference with my new Exude program is that this is one full hour of high intensity. The one hour that it takes me to do the Exude program is far more effective then the two hours that I used to spend at the gym before. I immediately started feeling my body changing! Not only was I able to do more cardiovascular work without getting as tired or running out of breath, but I also began feeling more energized during and after each workout.

I love the fact that I am able to work out with my mom; it makes each session all the more motivating and enjoyable. We both work out three days a week at Exude and three days on our own, and we are finally achieving the results that we have worked so hard for in the past. The most significant factor about the Exude program is that if you stick with it, the results occur. For about six months before I started working out at Exude, I had hit a plateau. I thought that I would never get the rest of the weight off. Not only was I unable to lose any more weight, I actually saw the scale starting to go up. After two months of working out at Exude, I have lost more weight and inches than I thought I would and could not be happier. When doing any kind of exercise, you only get out of it what you put into it. Exude's trainers and executive staff make it easy to stay focused and motivated. They have great attitudes and offer daily encouragement. I am psyched to continue working out hard and seeing more results the Exude way.

NAME: Heather Gallagher

DATE: December 12, 2002

AGE: 23

TOTAL INCHES LOST: 19

TOTAL WEIGHT LOST: 7 pounds

TIME IT TOOK TO LOSE THE WEIGHT: 6–8 months

PRIOR EXERCISE REGIMEN: I exercised a lot. I went to my gym and lifted heavy weights 4 days a week for my entire body. I also did cardio for 45 minutes on the elliptical machine 5 days a week.

CURRENT EXERCISE REGIMEN: I stick with my workout 3 days a week at Exude and do 3 days of the Exude prescribed off-day routines on my own, which include full upper- and lower-body exercises, calisthenics, abdominal work, jumping rope, and cardiovascular activity.

PRIOR EATING HABITS: I watched what I ate overall but was not consistent when it came to making the healthy choices I knew I should make. I cheated more than I should have and drank alcohol, which is very high in calories.

CURRENT EATING HABITS: I am trying to eat more varieties of foods with smaller portions, less snacking, and healthier choices during meals. I am also drinking less alcohol.

THE MAIN FACTOR THAT HELPED HEATHER TO ESCAPE HER WEIGHT: Since I started working out properly, I have seen great results each month. I know that all the hard work is paying off and that makes me more motivated to stick with eating healthy and exercising.

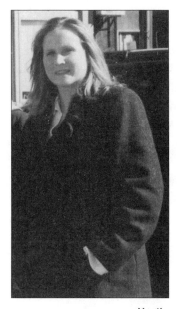 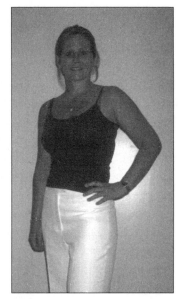

Heather Gallagher

Lallande de Gravelle—10 and Under Weight Loss

I did not come to this program looking for another quick fix. I had decided it was time for a total lifestyle change and was in search of a way to simplify my life *for the rest of my life*. Beyond cardio exercise, I was not very consistent with my workouts. I figured I would lose weight if I worked out hard aerobically—I thought that the harder and higher my resistance was during the aerobic portion of my exercise routine, the more calories I would burn. I would often try the "flavor-of-the-month" strength-training exercises that I read about in various fitness magazines. I knew that strength training was important; however, I never established a set routine, so I never stuck with anything and therefore I never saw results that equaled all the hard work I felt I was putting in.

After reading Edward's book and coming to Exude in New York City for an orientation session, I realized that I had to change my entire workout regimen. I am now *very* consistent with my exercise program and stick to six days per week no matter what. I do three days where my routine takes approximately 1¼ hours each and three days of approximately 1 hour each. My routines include warming up with cardio (recumbent bike—no resistance), stretching, jumping rope, a series of lower-and upper-body strength-training exercises (using a four-pound bar), and cooling down on the bike. Also, my routine now includes a whole series of advanced abdominal exercises that I have worked up to over time, pain, and a lot of sweat. The best part of all is that I have learned to do my abdominal routine with proper form, protecting my neck and lower back, and have excelled beyond just doing crunches. I even have a flat stomach for the first time. The core strength and flexibility I have developed has greatly improved my weekly ninety-minute yoga practice and energy level all day. I have discovered just how crucial it is to adhere to a consistent workout schedule as well as the importance of focusing on maintaining the correct form and control while performing all of the exercises. Even when the exercise seems next to impossible to continue doing (such as making it past five full sit-ups, which I thought I would never do—now I can do thirty-five!), I am aware that pushing myself to my personal limit and beyond is the only way I will continue seeing results.

In the past, I thought I knew how and what to do when it came to sticking with a healthy diet. I found that I could never maintain good habits long enough to see a change. I would get frustrated and try one diet or another sporadically as my weight would yo-yo, which frustrated me even more. I never really felt good on any of the diets that I tried and then I felt even worse when I realized that they had not worked.

I have realized that for me moderation is the key to keeping myself on track with a healthy diet/eating habits. I enjoy food far too much to make sacrifices required by many diets that are out there. However, I do find that since my body has changed and my energy level has increased, I now need to eat really well. I feel my best when I eat small amounts of wholesome food at regular intervals. And surprise, surprise, even my sweet tooth has diminished. I wish I had the willpower to totally eliminate my daily craving for a "sweet treat" (think small piece of cake, not the whole cake—moderation is the key!). I recognize that I could possibly achieve better results more quickly if I made this sacrifice. Since my goal is a lifestyle change, not a one-time fix, I chose to lose weight without foregoing those desserts and feeling deprived. I also knew that I would eventually return to my old "sugar" habit if I tried to eliminate it completely. Besides, I can certainly live with the results that I have achieved with my current diet, and I plan to continue and achieve all my long-term goals with my newfound Exude exercise routine.

NAME: Lallande de Gravelle
DATE: November 26, 2002
AGE: 33
TOTAL INCHES LOST: 14.25
TOTAL WEIGHT LOST: 10 pounds
TIME IT TOOK TO LOSE THE WEIGHT: 6 months
PRIOR EXERCISE REGIMEN:

- Elliptical machine (medium resistance) (30 minutes for 3 times/week)

- Lunges and squats (2 sets of 20 for each exercise) holding two five-pound weights (1–2 times/week)

- Yoga (1–2 times/week)

- Occasional upper body work (not consistent)

- No abdominal exercise (hurt neck and lower back too much)

CURRENT EXERCISE REGIMEN: I had been in search of a way to simplify my life and found the Exude program. I am *very* consistent with my exercise program, sticking to it six days per week. Three days a week I do a routine approximately 1¼ hour each; and three days I do another, which is approximately 1 hour each. My routines include a warm-up with cardio (recumbent bike—no resistance), stretching, jumping rope, a series of lower- and upper-body strength-training exercises for my hourglass figure (using a four-pound bar), and cooling down on the bike.

PRIOR EATING HABITS: I often tried to eat well and thought I knew how and what to do when it came to sticking with a healthy diet. I found that I could never maintain good habits long enough to see a change. I would get frustrated and try one diet or another and sporadically my weight would yo-yo, which frustrated me even more. I never really felt good on any of the diets that I tried, and then I felt even worse when I realized that they had not worked.

CURRENT EATING HABITS: Moderation is the key to my current eating habits. I enjoy food far too much and won't sacrifice by dieting. However, I do find that since my body has changed and my energy level has increased, I now need to eat really healthy. I feel my best when I eat small amounts of wholesome food at regular intervals. My sweet tooth has diminished. I recognize that I could possibly achieve better results more quickly if I cut sweets out altogether, but since my goal is a lifestyle change, not a one-time fix, I chose to lose weight without foregoing those desserts and feeling deprived.

THE MAIN FACTOR THAT HELPED LALLANDE TO ESCAPE HER WEIGHT: CONSISTENCY! CONSISTENCY! CONSISTENCY! Followed very, very closely by having perfect form and good control! I have learned how crucial it is to adhere to a consistent workout schedule as well as the importance of maintaining correct form while performing all exercises. Even when the exercise seems next to impossible to continue, I push myself to my limit and beyond so I will continue to see those results.

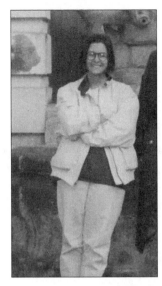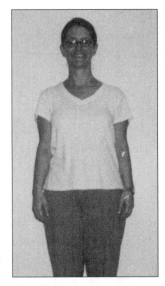

Lallande de Gravelle

Christine Gendreau—11–30 Weight Loss

You know the story. I'm sure you've heard one like it before or have a similar story yourself. I had shed about twenty pounds for my wedding and started eating at full speed on my honeymoon. By Christmas, I gained the twenty pounds I had lost plus about ten more.

When I tried to diet, my body was still in starvation mode from a deprivation diet I was on before my wedding, and it held on to everything I ate. My usual exercise routine was not working. I was exercising about five times a week, doing forty-five minutes of cardio and some weights. Nothing was happening, and I looked and felt worse and worse every day. I consoled myself with more food, telling myself I was just a happy newlywed and eventually I would stop eating so much.

I reached desperation when nothing in my closet fit. I went from a size 6 to a size 14 in about eight months. I bought new clothes, almost busting through a size 14 but determined to wear it since the next size was in another store altogether. In the fall, I wore skirts and tights to work so they held in my stomach. I was uncomfortable all day long at work as the tights dug into my body.

I was always uncomfortable with how my body was shaped; even when I lost weight, I was not really satisfied with how I looked. In my honeymoon pictures, my whole body looks pretty thin except for my stomach—that's where I gain weight first, and it's the last place for me to lose the weight. With a large waist that is not proportional to the rest of my body, it is impossible to find clothes that fit well, and I had always felt depressed because I looked bad in everything—especially pants! I dreamed of the day that I could wear jeans without being so self-conscious!

As I was pedaling away on my bike one morning, I saw Edward on *Today in New York* talking about Exude Fitness located in New York City. His theory made a lot of sense. Why couldn't I lose weight when I was exercising forty-five minutes five days a week? My metabolism, as well as my current fitness program needed a kick in the ass, and that's what it got when I hauled myself into Exude to meet with Lee Ross for my fitness assessment. Lee was really upbeat and encouraging. I did not feel embarrassed when she and Edward took what they said would be my "before" picture. I said that I wanted to increase my strength and try to get something I hadn't seen in a long time—a waist! They did not make me any false promises. They said if I just hung in there and kept with it, that I would see results.

The first few weeks I worked out about four times a week. I was finding the workouts much harder than my usual routine, but much more rewarding. I immediately felt energized after each workout. I hadn't worked up such a sweat since playing on a soccer team in the fifth grade! I felt that whatever I was doing must be working.

Gradually, the weight came off. Every few months I go back and work out at Exude with Lee. She takes measurements, offers encouragement, and tweaks my workouts up a notch. This is great, because I always have something to work up to, rather than doing the same exercise all the time! When I first started jumping rope, I could barely do fifty rotations. Now I am up to fifteen minutes!

It has been over a year now, and I still do the workouts four times a week. I'm now a 10—I look much better than I did at a size 6, if that makes sense. When I starved myself down to a 6, my body was not in proportion. But now, even though I weigh more than I did then, I am in much better proportion. Now I can wear pants! I have a closet full of pants, and I am no longer afraid to wear them!

I recently began following Weight Watchers so that I could get full control over my eating habits, which has helped me focus so much on what to eat and what *not* to eat, and I have lost more weight without feeling deprived.

Exude has been great. My only advice is to stick with it and you will see results! This is not a quick fix—it's a lifestyle change that will help you reshape your body, look and feel better about yourself, and become fit.

NAME: Christine Gendreau

DATE: November 19, 2002

AGE: 30

TOTAL INCHES LOST: 19.75

TOTAL WEIGHT LOST: 25 pounds

TIME IT TOOK TO LOSE THE WEIGHT: One year without serious dieting.

PRIOR EXERCISE REGIMEN: Bicycling 4 days a week at 45 minutes; weights 2 days a week.

CURRENT EXERCISE REGIMEN: Exude workout routines prescribed by Exude 4–5 days per week, which include a warm-up, jumping rope (a lot), calisthenics, abdominals, more jumping rope, stretching, a cooldown. I can do my routine at home before or after work and still fit in all the other things I need to get in weekly.

PRIOR EATING HABITS: Anything and everything in high volume

CURRENT EATING HABITS: I started following Weight Watchers, which is great for me, since they give you support. I still eat in high volume, but I make healthier choices and lately have been much better about my portion size.

THE MAIN FACTOR THAT HELPED CHRISTINE TO ESCAPE HER WEIGHT: Eating more healthy and having a support system as well as EXERCISE! EXERCISE! EXERCISE!

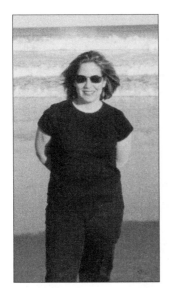 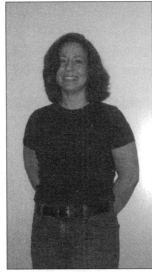

Christine Gendreau

Pam Utter—11–30 Weight Loss

While growing up, fitness or weight control was not the struggle it became later in life for me. For the first eighteen years of my life, I was a devoted dancer. I was taking as many as eight classes a week. I worked a part-time job and even cleaned the dance studios on Sundays in return for class tuition. At times it was a challenge, but there was no stopping me! I couldn't learn enough about dancing.

After pursuing a college education to establish a career as a court reporter, the focus and commitment I had always devoted to dance turned to mastering a new skill—a sedentary one—and that's where my body and self-image, as I knew it, started changing, and kept changing, for the worse.

Little did I know it would take the Escape Your Weight program to reclaim my body and myself as I once knew it and loved it. I wish I had found this program sooner!

During this gradual process of gaining weight, I was often a member of a gym but did not regularly work out. Deadlines at work were more important. My eating habits weren't as cautious as they should've been for not having an exercise program—not eating a balanced diet, let alone at normal hours of the day. The career and the deadlines always came first.

There were times when I would have a little success with a diet program or with starting a workout routine with a friend, but the results were never permanent. I just figured that this was my natural state and that I had better learn to accept it. Mother Nature was going to win this battle, sister. Get over it. The truth is, deep down, I refused to get over it. I would not be happy until I reclaimed myself.

After ten years of struggle and near surrender, it was obvious to me that I would need help in tackling this challenge. This was not a goal I could achieve on my own. I wanted to learn how to get my body back and live a healthier lifestyle. I was devoted, but I needed help. I had seen Edward on a television talk show discussing the Exude program, and I thought, *This has to work!* The program has different approaches for different types of people and challenges they may have and agrees with my philosophy that one size does *not* fit all.

Well, I called Exude Fitness and came in for my evaluation. I couldn't even do a sit-up without help. I was so upset at my "performance" I wanted to cry. I really didn't realize what I had done to myself over all these years. That didn't matter now; this was a showdown that I was going to win. I wasn't giving up. I started the program at Exude the next week. My trainer told me two things that I would need *every* time I worked out—commitment and intensity. As long as I had that, I couldn't fail. It wasn't long before I started to notice results and sit-ups were no longer a problem!

I have been following my Exude program for nearly three months, and my dream of reclaiming my body is coming true! In three months I have lost 35 inches and 20 pounds. I WIN! I *love* the way I feel now! I actually feel healthy. I am recognizing the body I am starting to see appear before my very eyes. I can fit into clothes I haven't in years (yes, I kept them), but best of all is how it feels when people say to me, "You look different; you're glowing!" This is a dream come true!

THANK YOU, ROBERT, and THANK YOU, EDWARD!! THANK YOU, EXUDE!!

NAME: Pamela Jane Utter

DATE: June 1, 2003

AGE: 34

TOTAL INCHES LOST: 35

TOTAL WEIGHT LOST: 20 pounds

TIME IT TOOK TO LOSE THE WEIGHT: 5 months

PRIOR EXERCISE REGIMEN: None, really.

CURRENT EXERCISE REGIMEN: Exude Fitness center and doing my homework on my own.

PRIOR EATING HABITS: Not a balanced diet and not at normal eating hours.

CURRENT EATING HABITS: Finding alternatives to "bad" foods and making sure I eat meals at better times in the day.

THE MAIN FACTOR THAT HELPED PAMELA TO ESCAPE HER WEIGHT: Finding the Exude program and sticking with it no matter how difficult it seems at times. It works for me: using it, learning it, and living it!

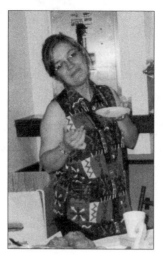
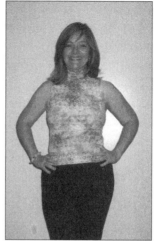

Pam Utter

Nancy Hsu—11–30 Weight Loss

As my senior year of high school headed toward its end, my worries switched from college admissions to what I was going to wear to the prom. In February, I made the decision to lose weight to look great for that upcoming night in June. My weight-loss plan included working out at least three days a week and consisted of an hour of cardio each day. I lost a few pounds by June and felt great, so I bought a new wardrobe to motivate myself to continue. Soon after that, I felt healthier and had more energy, but no matter how much exercise I did, I was unable to lose more weight. I needed a new approach to achieving the body I wanted and luckily came across New York City's Exude.com Fitness in a fashion magazine.

After much reading about Exude, I called and spoke to a woman named Lee Ross, who explained to me what I could expect on my first day; it seemed like the perfect solution for my situation, so I set up a fitness orientation with her at Exude. I decided that I would start a new life with the fitness guidance Exude had to offer me. I was assigned a trainer and was happy to see that after only a couple of sessions I was stronger and more flexible. My entire workout routine was changed and adapted to fit my needs and schedule. I had specific off-day workouts to do when I was not at Exude and wonderful challenging workouts when I was at Exude. Within two weeks I noticed that my clothes fit better and I was finally able to wear tiny tank tops without feeling at all self-conscious. Now it was the end of July, and I had lost a total of twenty pounds!

When it comes to eating, I make much better choices now and understand portion control and eating the right amounts of food that I know I will burn when I exercise. Something very important I learned at Exude is calories in verses calories out. I typically eat a good breakfast every morning, consisting of a bowl of Special K with a yogurt and sometimes a banana or a small low-fat bran muffin. Light lunches consist of a salad or a hummus wrap, and my dinner is usually steamed vegetables and a serving of pasta salad with some chickpeas *or* just another huge salad. I try to eat as little red meat as possible. I watch what snacks I eat during the day but especially after 8 P.M. My occasional snack is baked chips and once in a while Gummi bears.

I followed the Exude programs outlined for me throughout the rest of the summer and lost ten more pounds, a total of 12 inches, and have never felt better about myself. I have never jumped rope before Exude and now consider it the best and only tool I need to be physically fit. I enjoyed every session at Exude and am going to take everything I learned with me to college. In all, I have lost a total of thirty-pounds in about six months, and I plan to lose more since I now can work out the smart and right way for me.

NAME: Nancy Hsu

DATE: November 19, 2002

AGE: 18

TOTAL INCHES LOST: 12

TOTAL WEIGHT LOST: 30 pounds

TIME IT TOOK TO LOSE THE WEIGHT: 6 months

PRIOR EXERCISE REGIMEN: I exercised for about 5 months without seeing major results before going to Exude. I would do 10 minutes on the elliptical, then an hour or more of 2-minute intervals between level 10 and level 2 intensity. Sometimes after that I would hop on the bike for another 30 minutes of a cardio program. My exercise was mainly on the elliptical and was not a very healthy exercise program, as I was always there for more than two hours at a time. I didn't think I could continue doing that forever but was not sure what else to do to get results.

CURRENT EXERCISE REGIMEN: While at Exude, I did an Exude moderate to advanced full-body routine 4–5 times a week, which included: full-body routine, including jumping rope, calisthenics, and light resistance/high repetitions for upper and lower body, abdominal exercises. I have been back at school now since September 2002 and have accomplished one of my many goals: joining the women's rowing team. I continue with my Exude workout 2–3 times a week in addition to running 4 miles a day along with other strength training, cardio and working on the ergometer, and doing crew exercises similar to calisthenics called scullers': arms in, legs out, arms out, legs in, resting on butt, plus: Plyos: jumpies: jumping as high up in the air and getting butt all the way down to the ground, mountain climbers (I'm sure you know what these are, hands on ground, alternating feet back and forth), swimmers (stomach on floor, lifting quads up back and forth 30 seconds at a time), running stairs once a week (40 flights, 2 steps at a time), doing 6k ergometer tests once a week with an average split under 2 minutes and 25 seconds, as well as actually rowing in the boat.

PRIOR EATING HABITS: I was not very health-minded or educated about what to do before she started exercising and ate whatever and however much she wanted. When I started exercising I went to the other extreme and was very restrictive, cutting out all carbohydrates and eating only grilled chicken for every meal with an occasional fruit and/or vegetable. I was not sure how to modify or increase portions without getting hungry.

CURRENT EATING HABITS: I make much better choices now and understand portion control and eating the right amounts of food that I know I will burn when I exercise. I typically eat a good breakfast every morning consisting of a bowl of Special K with a yogurt and sometimes a banana or a small low-fat bran muffin. Light lunches consist of a salad or hummus wrap and dinner is usually steamed vegetables and a serving of pasta salad with some chickpeas or just another huge salad. I try to eat as little red meat as possible. I watch what snacks I eat during the day but especially after 8 P.M. My occasional snack is baked chips and once in a while Gummi bears.

THE MAIN FACTOR THAT HELPED NANCY TO ESCAPE HER WEIGHT: "Meeting with an Exude consultant three times a week and watching what I ate without depriving myself definitely helped me achieve my goals. I had amazing support and excitement from the Exude staff when I made improvements in my workout or in my weight/inch loss, which really motivated me to do better every time I did the workout."

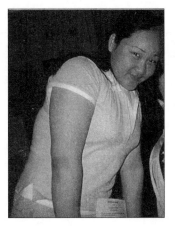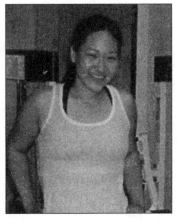

Nancy Hsu

Ellen Shurgan—11–30 Weight Loss

I have always tried to make exercise a part of my everyday life. I would attempt to plan a physical activity whenever I could. However, I would often find that weeks would go by and I did not find or make time to participate in the activity that I planned. I also tried to diet, beginning anew every Monday. Although I do not really pig out or eat very large portions, I enjoy good food and eating out often.

At one point, I even tried hiring a personal trainer at a local gym. Having an appointment did make me honor my commitment to exercise, but I found that my bottom half, always my trouble spot, seemed to be getting larger, rather than smaller. I was surprisingly bulking up in the exact places I needed to trim down. No matter how hard I worked, my shape was becoming even more exaggerated. I found this most discouraging and eventually stopped going to the gym altogether.

One day, while watching the *Morning Show* on Channel 4, I saw Jane Hanson at the Exude Fitness Center in Manhattan trying to reshape her body by losing unwanted inches. The segment caught my interest, since I was not tremendously overweight, but the weight was in all the wrong places. The segment addressed exercising correctly for your exact needs and lifestyle. They talked about how doing certain exercises could be harmful or helpful depending on the person. This really made sense to me, having seen firsthand how my exercise routine made me "bulk up."

I do not live in the city but decided to visit the Web site listed (exude.com). The site mentioned that you could visit the Exude Fitness facility and get a fitness assessment, resulting in a workout routine specifically designed for you. This program could be done at home without buying any major equipment, and I already owned a treadmill. It was such great news to know that I didn't even need to leave my house to start.

After the fitness assessment, I received my program and went home to begin performing it 3 days a week. It took me about a hour and a half at first. I played tennis one day a week and tried to walk about 3 miles outdoors on nice days. I found this exercise schedule very convenient. Within weeks, I began to notice results. My clothes fit better, and I had so much more energy. I really looked forward to exercising because it fit into my schedule so easily.

I did choose to make moderate changes to my diet. I began to eat three meals a day rather than skipping meals. I made sure to drink at least 6 eight-ounce glasses of water each day. I found the exercise program relieved stress, making me a lot happier and more energetic.

Finding Exude was a lifestyle change for me. I started the program in April 2002 and have continued to include it in my weekly activities. I went to visit the exercise studio twice to adjust the exercises slightly. Over the last year, I lost about 17 pounds and 28.25 inches, but how I look is not my major focus. Making healthy choices and taking care of my body for the rest of my life is the goal for me.

Exude has helped me to do this!!!

NAME: Ellen Shurgan

DATE: June 30, 2003

AGE: 48

TOTAL INCHES LOST: 28.25

TOTAL WEIGHT LOST: 17 pounds

TIME IT TOOK TO LOSE THE WEIGHT: 6 months

PRIOR EXERCISE REGIMEN: Gym, walking, tennis.

CURRENT EXERCISE REGIMEN: Making healthy lifestyle changes, which included adding my Exude prescribed exercise routine 3 times a week. Walk with my Exude homework plan 2 times a week, tennis once a week. Eating better meals.

PRIOR EATING HABITS: I skipped meals, didn't drink enough water, and didn't think about what I was eating.

CURRENT EATING HABITS: I plan my meals, don't skip any, and watch portions! I, of course, drink more water as well.

THE MAIN FACTOR THAT HELPED ELLEN TO ESCAPE HER WEIGHT: Making exercise and diet a part of my lifestyle. I plan to eat and exercise rather than diet!

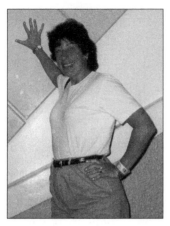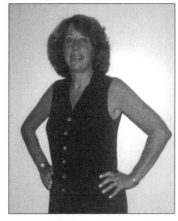

Ellen Shurgan

Carol Gallagher—11–30 Weight Loss

For as long as I can remember, if there was a diet or a weight program, I was the first in line with my credit card looking for the magic formula that would help me lose the weight. I have tried it all: weighing my food, having meals delivered to my house, new fad diets and those old diets that have been around for years. All that seemed to happen was that I would lose five pounds and then gain ten pounds. I didn't like what was happening to my body and found myself struggling mentally and physically. I stopped liking how I looked and after a while, I just didn't care. I continued to exercise at my gym with heavy weights and diet in spurts and ended up getting nowhere.

After never seeing results, I was frustrated and felt as though I failed. I became desperate and decided to have liposuction and a tummy tuck. This was against my principals; the thought of going under anesthesia gave me anxiety. To this day, I still can't believe I went through with it, but at the time, I thought it was the only way to get rid of the unwanted weight and inches. It ended up being just another quick fix. The weight came back on again.

One day my daughter was reading the paper and saw an article about Exude Fitness located in New York City. She immediately was interested in the program and their unique methodology and wanted me to go check it out with her. I was apprehensive about going, thinking it would be yet another program promising results and not delivering. I amused her and went in for the fitness assessment and was pleasantly surprised by the routine we were put through. It was very different from anything either of us had done in the past and that made me think maybe this might finally work. I live two hours from the city and had to consider whether traveling was something I wanted to commit to. I realized that if this program worked, it would be well worth all the travel time, so I decided to give it a try.

I started doing the workouts and noticed quick results, which brought my motivation level to an all-time high. Thanks to my daughter, I now look forward to working out and feel as though it is no longer a chore but something I really enjoy. The results are remarkable! I have been doing the Exude program for about eight months and have lost a total of 47.50 inches and 29 pounds. My clothes fit better, and most of all, I feel better about myself inside and out.

I am looking forward to losing more inches and weight and reaching all my long-term goals. I know that with this program it will happen. In hindsight, I would never have gone for liposuction if I had know I could do it the Exude way. Working out with my daughter is a challenge because she pushes me past what I would do on my own. My Exude workout is so much more efficient and manageable than going to the gym and using the equipment the wrong way and hurting myself. Never again will I pick up those heavy weights and rack them on and off the machines.

Thank you, Exude!!!

NAME: Carol Gallagher

DATE: December 12, 2002

AGE: 47

TOTAL INCHES LOST: 47.50

TOTAL WEIGHT LOST: 29 pounds

TIME IT TOOK TO LOSE THE WEIGHT: 8 months

PRIOR EXERCISE REGIMEN: I did a heavy weight-lifting routine for my entire body. I would break up body parts and add a little cardio now and then.

CURRENT EXERCISE REGIMEN: I exercise 5 days a week–2 days at Exude and 3 days at home on my Exude off-day program, one of which is more cardiovascular and the other is more of a full-body workout.

PRIOR EATING HABITS: I ate whatever I wanted and did not make the healthiest choices. I dined at restaurants a lot, which made it difficult to control the way food was prepared and the portion size. I also tried many different diets and weight-loss tricks.

CURRENT EATING HABITS: I make an effort to eat much healthier now overall. I prepare my own meals and make better choices when I do go out to a restaurant.

THE MAIN FACTOR THAT HELPED CAROL TO ESCAPE HER WEIGHT: Being consistent with my prescribed exercise program, seeing results helped me stay on track and be committed as well as eating much healthier daily.

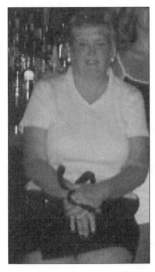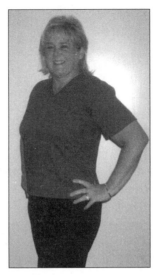

Carol Gallagher

Lynn Leff—11–30 Weight Loss

Approximately three years ago I became so frustrated with my weight and began running on the treadmill five days per week. Despite my exercise choice and commitment, there was no change in my body or my weight. I hated the way my body looked, especially in my arms.

After coming into work day after day and expressing this frustration to my coworking friend, she sent me an e-mail about Exude, and it got me interested. Maybe it was perfect timing or my increasing frustration that made me pick up the phone and book my first appointment at Exude. I am so happy that I did because it has changed my outlook and attitude on fitness, not to mention what it has done for my figure.

I have had successful and satisfying results by continuing my Exude training on my own and working out at home on the Exude program and watching my food intake with Weight Watchers. I have lost weight and inches and went from a size 10 to a size 6. When it comes to achieving and maintaining results, Exude has the winning combination!

The results have been tremendous, but the Exude environment has been such a motivating factor in my realization that exercise can be enjoyable and beneficial for the rest of my life! The Exude staff deserves mentioning; from the receptionist to the owner you are treated with warmth and as a part of their family. This place is awesome, and the knowledge I now possess because of Exude has made an incredible difference in my life.

Sincerely,

Lynn Leff

NAME: Lynn Leff

DATE: December 9, 2002

AGE: 48

TOTAL INCHES LOST: 14

TOTAL WEIGHT LOST: 15 pounds

TIME IT TOOK TO LOSE THE WEIGHT: 9 months

PRIOR EXERCISE REGIMEN: I was not consistent with any program. I started running on the treadmill three times a week sometime before joining Exude and had not seen or felt any results. I mainly focused on exercising and not watching my food intake. I thought that if I was exercising, I could pretty much eat what I wanted.

CURRENT EXERCISE REGIMEN: I exercise three to five times a week. I now do all of my workouts on my own at home.

PRIOR EATING HABITS: I never watched how many carbohydrates I ate or controlled my portion size.

CURRENT EATING HABITS: I have learned that I definitely need to watch what I eat. I joined Weight Watchers and now watch my portion size.

THE MAIN FACTOR THAT HELPED LYNN TO ESCAPE HER WEIGHT: The Exude workouts really made a difference in how I felt about myself. I was motivated to continue and felt good. I saw some results in my body but knew that I would need to change my diet to really lose inches and weight. The combination of the right nutrition adjustments and a consistent exercise program got me to reach my goals and stay motivated.

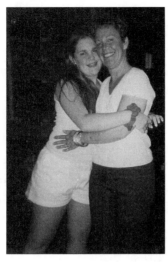
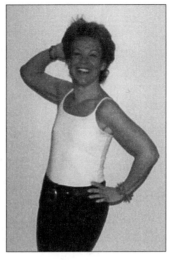

Lynn Leff

Barbara Bacci Mirque—11–30 Weight Loss

I am not one of those people who tried every diet book on the market. I considered myself too intelligent to look for a silver bullet and smart enough to know the basics—that I had to eat right, choose moderate portions, and exercise. Despite my supposed intelligence, I carried around an extra twenty pounds for years and years. I would lose weight on sensible diets such as Weight Watchers (and getting married for the first time at 46 was too nervous to even diet!) then gain it back. My body set point was 145 pounds (give or take a few pounds), and I would get below 140 then go right back to 145 when I stopped being vigilant. And by the way, exercise was never an integral part of my diet routine—I would add exercise in spurts, and I know now usually incorrect ones such as step classes and exercising at home on my stair-climbing machine was wrong. And I admit I was a tad lazy, too, not to mention the fact that I have a classic curvy shape, which means I could carry more weight than people would ever guess.

However, as I unabashedly approached fifty, I vowed that looking and feeling healthy were paramount. As a classic self-absorbed baby boomer, I want to fight aging with every bone in my body, and carrying around extra weight doesn't help, nor does it help one look younger! I started a fabulous job two and a half years ago with a commute into Manhattan of an hour and a half each way from my home in suburban New York. A year into the commute—a little over a year and a half ago—I complained to my husband that I had no time to exercise and it was all his fault because we live near his business. He was sweet enough to take the abuse and not point out that I had not been exercising that much before I started this job. That same morning my husband happened to see Edward Jackowski, Ph.D., on *The Early Show*, and primarily to shut me up I am sure, he looked up the program and e-mailed me the Exude Web site information. I called that day, set up an appointment with Edward on Valentine's Day 2002, and signed up on the spot as a Valentine's Day present to myself.

During my first meeting with Edward, he said a few things that frightened me and a few things about which I was skeptical. First, what frightened me was that he said I would never weigh less than 130 pounds (forget the fact I weighed over 140 pounds and I wanted to weigh 115!); I would have to exercise five times a week to lose weight and three times a week to maintain my weight, and I would learn to like to jump rope! I did not have the time to add exercise at that rate, so this was never going to work I replied, and the jump rope was for kids. I was very skeptical when he said his program worked—how many times had I heard that from every quack peddling diet pills on television?! However, a few things caught my attention when we went through a sample routine. I think I instinctively knew that Edward's approach was practical and based on sound principles, and I knew I needed someone and something to jump start me on the road to physical fitness and a better shape. I liked that Edward said you don't need a gym or fancy athletic equipment. And he also said stop thinking you have to weigh some magic number (115) that you will never achieve. Instead, he said, "I am going to make you look as if you weigh 115." That struck a chord. If he could pull that off, and he said he could, then I wanted in!

The result: I do not weigh 115, but I do wear a size 4 or 6 (and I even bought two pairs of a size 2 Ann Taylor stretch pants that fit like a dream!) because my waist, hips, thighs, and calves have all been whittled down. My old "skinny" jeans that I used to squeeze myself into as a measure of how thin I was became too big and have long since been given away. I look better than I ever have in my life.

Now I have a sleek red tank dress that I am going to wear on my fiftieth birthday. And by the way, exercise and eating right is part of my life, especially jumping rope! Fifty will be my best decade ever!!!! Thanks, Exude, for starting me on the path to fitness and my best shape.

NAME: Barbara Bacci Mirque
DATE: March 18, 2003
AGE: 49
TOTAL INCHES LOST: 15.75

TOTAL WEIGHT LOST: 14 pounds

TIME IT TOOK TO LOSE THE WEIGHT: 4 months

PRIOR EXERCISE REGIMEN: I enjoyed being active, and I ski, hike, and sail, but I had never exercised consistently. From time to time I would get into exercise spurts and attend aerobic or step classes or join a health club and use their equipment (most likely incorrectly), but I did not remain with any program on an ongoing basis. Years ago, I purchased a stair climber (since banned from my house!) thinking it would be easier to exercise at home, and again, I would go through spurts of using that equipment, then abandon it to gather dust. I enjoy walking and would try to walk when the weather was nice but not at a high-intensity level. Needless to say, when I first joined Exude, I was not very physically fit, although I probably would have rated myself as so.

CURRENT EXERCISE REGIMEN: Finding Exude through a serendipitous confluence of events and growing to enjoy exercising. Scheduling my Exude workouts the same way I would a business appointment. I work out with my hunky Exude instructor twice a week (three times, if I can fit it in but that does not happen too often) and follow my off-day and on-day routines at home 2–3 times more a week. If I travel, I follow my Exude travel routine and take my jump rope with me. I look forward to traveling because the time I would have spent commuting is spent exercising in a hotel gym! I must tell you I hated to jump rope in the beginning, but now I look forward to it. I also purchased a stationary bike, and both my husband and I use that quite a bit!

PRIOR EATING HABITS: I would try to watch what I ate but was not really monitoring my portion sizes. Although I started eating healthier after my wedding in January 2000 because my husband cooks and he only uses fresh ingredients (I was eating lots of Lean Cuisines and/or cheerios/cheese and crackers dinners prior to getting married), I started to eat the same portion sizes as he did. I would eat cookies and cakes when they were served at meetings, parties, or restaurants without really thinking about how much I was eating.

CURRENT EATING HABITS: I control my portions, record what I eat, and am a bit more conscious of trade-offs. For example, I know if I have that glass of wine or two with dinner, then I must cut out something else. Recording what I eat, even after the fact, has really made me conscious of my eating habits, portion sizes, what I need to modify, and what I need to eliminate. On the days I exercise, I can eat a bit more, but since I still want to lose some weight, I try to use my exercise days to decrease my total weekly caloric intake. I have a sweet tooth but will restrict sweets to when we are out of the house, so there are no leftovers around to tempt me. I do like good, crusty artisan bread but am more conscious about the need to serve bread with dinner on a limited basis. Lastly and most importantly, I don't beat myself up should I over indulge or use "blowing my diet" as an excuse to binge. Rather, I try to add an extra exercise routine to burn off some of those extra calories.

THE MAIN FACTOR THAT HELPED BARBARA TO ESCAPE HER WEIGHT: The main factor is following an exercise regimen that is tailor-made to me and my strength level. The other thing I do now is I schedule my Exude workouts the same way I would schedule a business appointment. As far as my routine, as I continue to get stronger and stronger, Edward increases the intensity of my workout, so that I keep making progress instead of reaching a plateau. We all know that a consistent exercise routine is one of the keys of weight loss and subsequent weight control, but it is also not just how often you exercise but what you do and at what intensity level. From a diet standpoint, I did not diet, rather I monitored my intake and outtake of calories and attempted to eat at the caloric level at which I would lose weight. For example, on my sedentary office-only days, I applied Edward's slug formula (ten times your current weight) to determine the number of calories to eat and still lose weight and on my Exude workout days, I either could eat the same amount of calories and lose weight a bit faster or eat a bit more due to the increased activity level and still lose weight. Having the ability to "work off" my favorite foods enabled me to never feel deprived or on a "diet."

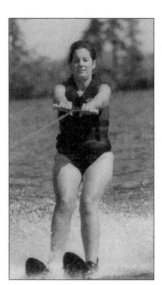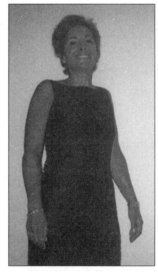

Barbara Bacci Mirque

Carol Turner—11–30 Weight Loss

I had never exercised consistently, although I knew I should have. I reached a very unfit and unhealthy point in my life and knew I needed to do something drastic. In the past, I would get excited and follow the latest exercise craze or fad that touted it was going to give me those quick healthy results that I craved. I joined almost every health club in the city for a couple months to a year and would actually only go a few times and then give up on myself again.

I discovered Exude Fitness in Manhattan and their philosophy immediately captured my attention. After my first day at Exude, I knew I could stick with it. It was a convenient distance from work and home, and I had a great support system in them, not to mention that I started looking and feeling better within weeks. The quick results motivated me to stick with the program while I was at home, and I managed to add an additional day per week with ease. I make a conscious effort to be consistent with my exercise routine and allow myself to be challenged by my Exude fitness consultant without getting frustrated.

I have lost over 9 inches in 20.50 pounds and continue to find it easy to keep up with the Exude workouts. I have committed to making healthier choices when it comes to my meals and snacks. I never have to deprive myself as long as I stick with my weekly workouts, and to top it off, I am never bored. The workout routines have allowed me to vary my exercises, try new things, and sharpen my athletic skills. I look forward to more amazing results and the continued inches dropping off!

Thanks,

Carol Turner

DATE: May 29, 2003

AGE: 49

TOTAL INCHES LOST: 9.00

TOTAL WEIGHT LOST: 20.50 pounds

TIME IT TOOK TO LOSE THE WEIGHT: 5 to 7 months

PRIOR EXERCISE REGIMEN: Every now and then I would follow the latest exercise craze. I joined almost every health club for a year and would only go for about two months of that time. I am the health club's "best friend."

CURRENT EXERCISE REGIMEN: I found the Exude Fitness center in Manhattan and after my first day received terrific encouragement from the Exude personnel to stick with the program. After I saw results, it got easier and the personal support never ceased. I exercise twice a week at Exude and do my off-day routine once a week at home. My job as a law firm administrator managing two offices in two parts of the city actually keeps me physically active on a daily basis.

PRIOR EATING HABITS: I rarely ate anything "green," and when I'd walk into my neighborhood coffee shop, I never had to order—the waiters knew to bring over my usual cheeseburger and fries.

CURRENT EATING HABITS: I enjoy a salad for lunch most weekdays. When eating out, I really look at what I'm eating regarding the size of the portion and generally find I don't have to eat the whole meal before I'm full. I have found it's okay not to "clean my plate" as my mother always had instructed.

THE MAIN FACTOR THAT HELPED CAROL TO ESCAPE HER WEIGHT: Making a conscious effort to follow an exercise routine on a consistent basis beneficial to my specific needs, fitness level, and lifestyle. Having a constant awareness of what I ate and what I didn't eat.

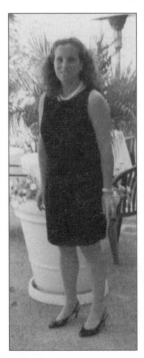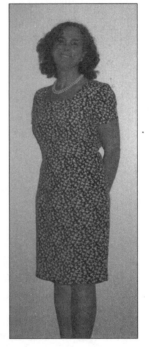

Carol Turner

Robert Lazarus—31–60 Weight Loss

First, let me start off by thanking all the Exude executives. I came to Exude looking for a job, and it was the best move I ever made in my life. Since I read Edward's book, I have worked hard to change my body by incorporating the right exercises into my workout regimen. I have always gained muscle mass easily. I used to go to the gym and lift heavy weights without warming up and stretching beforehand or cooling down when I was finished with my workout. I continued to get bigger and more muscular even though my goal was to cut up the muscles I already had and decrease some of my mass.

When I started working out I weighed 240 pounds and was inflexible and tight. Edward prescribed an exercise program for me, and I began seeing results quickly. I lost forty pounds in three months. I used to think I could eat what I wanted when I wanted it but that is just not true. The more I ate, the more mass I kept on my body, so I changed my eating habits around and cut out my carbohydrate intake after 6 P.M. I eat more vegetables and of course a lot of protein all day. I know it is hard to believe, but it is a year and half later and I have kept the weight off by continuing with the Exude program and watching what I eat and how much I work out. It has become a part of my life forever.

Thank you, Exude.

NAME: Robert Lazarus

DATE: December 12, 2002

AGE: 35

TOTAL INCHES LOST: n/a

TOTAL WEIGHT LOST: 40 pounds

TIME IT TOOK TO LOSE THE WEIGHT: 4–5 months

PRIOR EXERCISE REGIMEN: I would stick to a heavy weight-lifting routine for my entire body, splitting up my upper- and lower-body on different days. The workout was done at low-intensity and took me longer than I would have liked it to, but I thought that was what I had to do to keep myself strong. I didn't do a warm-up, and I rarely ever stretched before or after. I continued to get bigger and more muscular, even though my goal was to reduce some of my mass and get leaner.

CURRENT EXERCISE REGIMEN: I start with a warm-up, then a full-body stretch. I go on to my workload, which includes using light weights or a light-weighted bar for my entire upper body. I do pull-ups, chins and dips, and, of course, push-ups. My workouts are done at a fast pace and at a high intensity. I do a 3–5 minute cooldown at the end of every workout. I also jump rope two days a week for about 40–50 minutes and two days a week on my off-day. I also box.

PRIOR EATING HABITS: I would eat bigger portions one or two times a day and a lot of carbohydrates anytime of the day and more than I was burning off during my workouts.

CURRENT EATING HABITS: I eat a lot of different types of food and don't say the word NO when it come to eating what I want or crave. Instead of eating one or two bigger meals during the day, I try to eat smaller meals a few times a day and cut out eating carbohydrates after 6 P.M.

THE MAIN FACTOR THAT HELPED ROBERT TO ESCAPE HIS WEIGHT: The main factor was definitely making the changes to my workout to fit my needs. I do much more cardio, light weights, and more repetitions with high intensity. If I feel like I need to burn a few extra calories, I jump rope one extra day for 30 or 40 minutes.

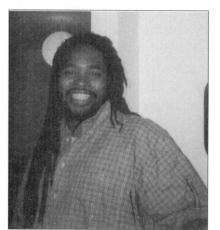 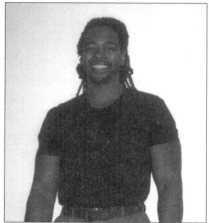

Robert Lazarus

Laura Goldzung—31–60 Weight Loss

For over 15 years, I rode the roller coaster of weight gain and loss. I experimented with a variety of diet programs and exercise regimes; yet, each year I was a bit heavier than the last. I would often see photos of myself and could not reconcile that I was the same person who looked back in my mirror each morning. Over time, I went from being very active in martial arts to becoming sedentary and suffering from chronic back pain. When my chiropractor suggested that my pain would be reduced by 85 percent if my weight were reduced by 30 percent, I had an epiphany! Always the optimist, I motivated myself to be motivated—in other words, I did everything conceivable to further motivate myself. I joined Weight

Watchers online. I went to the gym. I purchased one of Edward's informercial products as well as became a client of Exude's Personal Training Fitness Center in New York City. I listened to hypnotherapy tapes and to Tony Robbins. I read *Shape* magazine, *Self* magazine, and every other publication applicable to positive change and inner motivation.

The key lesson learned in the last 15 years is that you won't accomplish a goal until you are emotionally and intellectually ready to do so. It's a matter of self-leadership, and while I am still a work in progress, I'm already there mentally. I've reached my initial weight loss goal and look forward to it continuing!

NAME: Laura Goldzung

DATE: March 25, 2003

AGE: 50

TOTAL INCHES LOST: n/a

TOTAL WEIGHT LOST: 32 pounds

TIME IT TOOK TO LOSE THE WEIGHT: 5 months

PRIOR EXERCISE REGIMEN: Stop and start method—treadmill/bike/stretch

CURRENT EXERCISE REGIMEN: A full-body exercise regimen, including muscle toning and cardio in a circuit format—doing it right for long-lasting results.

PRIOR EATING HABITS: Consisted of fad dieting, too many refined carbs, and buying into the no-fat lifestyle.

CURRENT EATING HABITS: I am following a balanced and healthy nutrition program to achieve weight loss and reasonable lifetime eating habits.

THE MAIN FACTOR THAT HELPED LAURA TO ESCAPE HER WEIGHT: Getting motivated and staying motivated with a program that made sense to me and worked within my lifestyle.

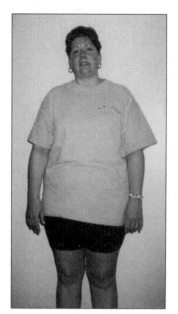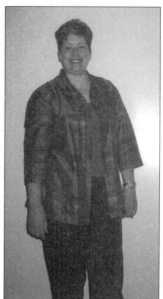

Laura Goldzung

Heather Passaro—31–60 Weight Loss

I'm sitting at my computer, and it's summer-in-the-city. Hot, humid, sticky, and irritating. I just got laid-off from my job and I'm depressed, not so much about losing my job—after all, this is New York City; you can always get another job. It was more about the fact that here was another summer and I was overweight. In fact, I was very overweight, and it was getting physically uncomfortable and I knew I might also be endangering my health.

In California, where I grew up, if you have time off with unemployment benefits you do what all California girls do: You check the want ads on Sunday, mail out your résumés on Monday, and wait it out for the rest of the week at the beach while working on your tan. Well, this was New York City and getting to the surf and sand is complicated and the thought of wanting to work on a tan to look fit and healthy in a size 18 bathing suit from the chubby girls' department at Lord & Taylor wasn't exactly appealing! That was it; I couldn't go through the rest of my life this way. I had to fix my problem, but I couldn't do it with food. Diets had never worked for me. In fact, my sister snapped at me on the phone, "Heather, you're the worst dieter." It may have been a passing comment, but something about her tone was more like a slap. I took it to mean that my friends and family don't take me seriously. I had to switch my focus off of food and find another way to lose the unwanted weight and inches.

I was logging onto my computer ready to search for my next job and there was this flash on my AOL home page: *Learn How Miss Universe Lost All Her Weight! Donald Trump Employs Exude Fitness in NYC to Trim Down Chubby Beauty*. I was curious and gave Exude a call. I didn't want to lose my focus. I heard myself ask, "Can I come in right now?" That was the first day of my journey back to a more balanced body, mind, and spirit.

I shower, blow dry my hair, and do my makeup, and for what? "You're going to work out, silly, and it's the middle of August; you're going to look like a melted grilled cheese sandwich when you get there." I ignore myself. I head up on the subway to midtown with my workout clothes and sneakers. One of Exude's program directors puts me through a fitness assessment/workout. "This is not a gym; it's a fitness center," he tells me. Cool! Here's my Amex. I had made a commitment of some serious money. What was Ira, my significant other, going to say? What could he say? "Honey, I love you just the way you are." Maybe he does, but modern psychology teaches us "you have to love yourself before anyone else can love you." So I explained to him it had nothing to do with money but was about self-love.

It's now been nearly two years and I have been exercising and eating healthier thanks to the common sense life-long approach that Exude has taught me. Aside from now being fit for the first time in my life, I look and feel twenty years younger. I am extremely healthy and fit and know that I will stick with this program for the rest of my life.

NAME: Heather Passaro

DATE: November 14, 2002

AGE: 46

TOTAL INCHES LOST: 55.50

TOTAL WEIGHT LOST: 57 pounds

TIME IT TOOK TO LOSE WEIGHT: 1 year

PRIOR EXERCISE REGIMEN: No prior exercise history

CURRENT EXERCISE REGIMEN: I perform my Exude full-body routine 3 times per week for 60 minutes, including stationary biking, jumping rope, calisthenics, abdominal exercises, light weights/high repetitions for both upper and lower body. I do mainly aerobic exercises and abdominal exercises for 50 minutes 2 times per week for my off-day routine.

PRIOR EATING HABITS: I had poor eating habits. I ate large portions of whatever I wanted. I would attempt extreme diets now and then and lose a little and then gain it back.

CURRENT EATING HABITS: I eat almost everything I want, but in moderation. I am more conscious of limiting starchy foods, especially at night. I snack less on junk food, and I make healthier choices.

THE MAIN FACTOR THAT HELPED HEATHER TO ESCAPE HER WEIGHT: I realized that here was another summer, and I was still overweight. In fact, I was very overweight, and it was getting physically uncomfortable for me to do the day-to-day things I needed to do. I also knew that I was endangering my health, and that scared me. I wanted to look fit and healthy! When I went shopping and realized that I would have to buy a size 18 bathing suit from the chubby girls' department at Lord & Taylor, that was it! I couldn't go through the rest of my life this way. I had to fix my problem. Enter Exude. Thank you to all at Exude.

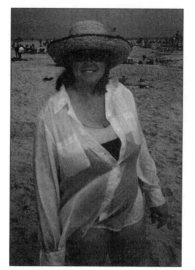 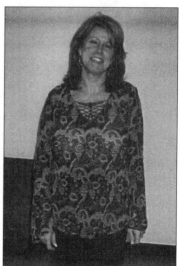

Heather Passaro

Dabee Kaye—31–60 Weight Loss

I have struggled with my weight my entire life. I can remember as a child being chunkier than all my friends and being frustrated even then. I tried every diet I could, in addition to having an eating disorder, but none of them worked. If I did have any success on a program, I always gained the weight back. I have also been diagnosed with a hypothyroid, so my weight loss is much slower than most. My life became a roller coaster of weight-loss programs and diets.

I had gotten to a point where I had come to terms with my weight and that I would be heavy forever. I wasn't happy about it, but I didn't know what else to do. Then an opportunity presented itself, and I decided to take advantage of it, instead of sitting on my couch and thinking about it six months after the fact. I met with Edward, and he explained to me that I could lose weight and change my body and that he had the tools to make that happen. I decided I needed to trust him and see what happened. Well, I have to tell you it wasn't easy and still isn't easy, but I look like a different person.

The first time I worked out with him I could only jump rope twenty-five jumps. Now I am up to about ten minutes with breaks, and that feels great. I still have the motivation to continue and love that feeling. I notice that my mindset has changed, and sometimes I find myself taking a walk or at the gym instead of eating. I am losing weight slower than others, so I need to be patient, but the weight is coming off and I am getting healthier in the meantime.

The one thing I never tried was a consistent exercise program that was right for me. I can honestly say it works and does wonders. I still have a ways to go, but being able to see the results now only continues to motivate me for the future. I have friends that are now on the program because they have seen my results, and they are doing great, too! I recommend this program and thank everyone at Exude for their support and encouragement.

NAME: Dabee Kaye

DATE: June 3, 2003

AGE: 30

TOTAL INCHES LOST: 30

TOTAL WEIGHT LOST: 33 pounds

TIME IT TOOK TO LOSE THE WEIGHT: 7 months

PRIOR EXERCISE REGIMEN: Kickboxing and yoga. I had never been consistent with exercise. I would go through spurts of taking classes or doing programs but never stuck to anything. My friends always tried to get me to go to a class with them, and some succeeded but others didn't. If it wasn't convenient and easy, I didn't make the time for it.

CURRENT EXERCISE REGIMEN: I train at Exude two days a week and work out on average three days a week at my gym. I typically do thirty minutes of cardio, stretch, jump rope, and do my abs and arms workout. When I travel, I take my jump rope with me and stay at hotels that have a gym.

PRIOR EATING HABITS: I watched what I ate but not closely. I definitely ate more bread and starches. If I was in a rush, I would grab a hamburger or something from a fast-food restaurant. I did a lot of take-out and didn't really take the time to look at what was in the food I was ordering.

CURRENT EATING HABITS: I still watch what I eat, but I am now aware of what goes in my body and why. I still eat breads and starches, but I now eat brown rice, wheat bread, and I limit my intake. I also rarely eat fast food and choose to grab salads instead of hamburgers. I still get take-out, but sauces are on the side or my choices are better.

THE MAIN FACTOR THAT HELPED DABEE TO ESCAPE HER WEIGHT: I got to a point in my life where I knew I had to do something. I was given an opportunity to meet Edward and learn about his program. I knew it couldn't hurt to try another program and thought this might actually work, since nothing had in the past. Within the last seven months I have watched my body change and essentially shrink. My clothes don't fit, and I feel better. This is only the beginning for me. I can't imagine what is to come, but I'm excited to see the results.

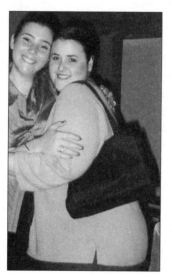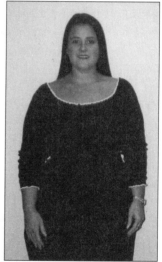

Dabee Kaye

Marlene Botter—31–60 Weight Loss

I've lost weight before—three other times in the past twenty years and always a loss of thirty pounds or more. But each weight loss was achieved through various diets—some of them drastic—that were never really integrated into my lifestyle on a long-term basis. I was an overweight child from a sedentary family with a food heritage that includes tons of simple carbs and fat-heavy preparation. Back in the days of "a fat baby is a healthy baby," I never could "eat just one" and was often encouraged to eat more.

When I would achieve my goal weight in the past, I never seemed able to maintain it beyond a few months. In my early twenties, I lost a lot of weight by drinking tea throughout the day and having just one meal a day, dinner. In my early thirties, I miraculously came away from a car accident requiring only eight weeks of my jaw wired shut and meals by straw. The forced fast left me slim but not toned. Subsequently, I threw myself into step classes with a vengeance and managed to reach an elite athlete's level of fitness. Not being able to sustain that rigor while also establishing my career, it wasn't long before my weight started its uphill climb. Fast forward to late thirties, another forty-five-pound weight loss, this time on one of those prepared foods diets, where the portions seemed too tiny for my large 5'8" frame. I was always hungry.

Once again, my weight crept upwards during a time when my work required me to travel weekly for months at a time, which meant restaurant meals at least four nights per week. Once the travel subsided, most food choices were based on convenience and included lots of processed and packaged foods. Also, by this time, I had enough information to acknowledge that I was a binge eater, and I needed help. My social activities had drastically cut back. I hated to shop for clothes because I was now in a size that shamed me, and the negative self-talk was nonstop.

I started doing research and after many months of pondering whether to invest in a personal trainer, I chose Exude. I'll never forget my first workout with my trainer. Thank goodness I sweat so much; it masked the tears I shed. I was so deeply disappointed at myself for allowing my fitness level to slip so far. But in a short time, I began to feel the benefits of my Exude sessions: My flexibility and strength increased. I was handling stress better and sleeping better. After six months, I discovered that I was finally looking forward to my training session and was motivated to exercise on my own consistently, but I had not reached my weight-loss goals. That's when I started researching nutrition. I picked a nutrition plan that spoke to all the food challenges I was juggling: carb cravings, chaotic schedule, and the impact of stress on cortisol levels, among others. During my research, I also discovered Internet support groups I could participate in. Bottom line: You've got to deal with your stuff; that baggage doesn't empty itself!

I've found this three-pronged approach of diet, exercise, and emotional support to work for me. Since I have focused on all of my challenges, I've lost 50 pounds and 30 inches. Imagine how much easier jumping rope has become! I've learned exercises I can continue to do when I travel. Most important, I'm learning to integrate balance, moderation, and consistency. I feel better about myself. I have every confidence that I'll not only reach my goal weight, but I have a firm grasp on the tools that will help me keep my overall fitness and health throughout my entire life.

NAME: Marlene Botter

DATE: May 26, 2003

AGE: 41

TOTAL INCHES LOST: 24.50

TOTAL WEIGHT LOST: 50 pounds

TIME IT TOOK TO LOSE THE WEIGHT: 10 months

PRIOR EXERCISE REGIMEN: None

CURRENT EXERCISE REGIMEN: Twice-weekly trainer-led workouts at Exude. An additional two to three days per week of either: yoga or Pilates videos, recumbent bike, walking, or Exude off-day program, followed by 15–20 minutes of jump rope.

PRIOR EATING HABITS: My weight crept upwards during a time when my work required me to travel weekly for long periods of time, which meant restaurant meals at least 4 nights per week. Once the travel subsided, most food choices were based on convenience and included lots of processed and packaged foods. I also struggled with a binge eating disorder.

CURRENT EATING HABITS: Four months ago, I began following a liver-supportive, fat-loss nutrition plan (Fat Flush Plan). I eat a balance of proteins, essential fats, and complex carbohydrates five times throughout day and do NOT eat sugar, salt, white or processed starches, wheat, dairy, caffeine, trans fats nor alcohol.

THE MAIN FACTOR THAT HELPED MARLENE TO ESCAPE HER WEIGHT: I turned to the Exude experts for help when I couldn't do it on my own.

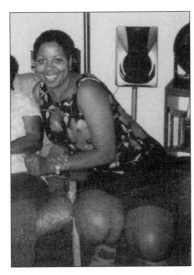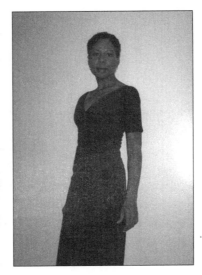

Marlene Botter

Ann Marie Curd-Fruhauf—31–60 Weight Loss

I have been struggling with my weight all of my life and, like many people, was always looking for the next great instantaneous miracle weight-loss program. It was always the same story. I would promise myself to go on a diet and would start with the best of intentions. I would, of course, join a gym to try and expedite the process. Finally, after a few weeks of seemingly endless two-hour-plus workouts and depriving myself of food, I would give up my newly found regimen, having achieved minimal results. To make matters worse, my workouts at the gym did not do much for decreasing my circumference. If anything, the parts I wanted to deemphasize usually got bigger.

One evening I was wandering around a book store, and Dr. Jackowski's book *Escape Your Shape* caught my eye. I swore that I would never throw away money on another book about fitness or diet, but after walking by it several times, I couldn't help but pick it up and skim through it. The philosophy of the book made so much sense to me that I broke my rule and bought it. I figured I would give it a try. I had nothing to lose except the unwanted weight and inches.

I needed a piece of equipment for the workout that I could not find anywhere, so I looked in the book to find a number or Web site for Exude. To my surprise, Exude was not only located in New York City but was across the street from my office. I went over that evening after work with the intention of buying a piece of exercise equipment; I came out with an appointment for an evaluation and initial workout.

After my initial session, I told myself that I would do what they say, give it a few weeks, and see where it went. The whole theory sounded good, but would it work? I admit I wasn't too optimistic, given my past track record. But after only a few weeks, I could see a difference. I could not believe how my body was changing. I was getting stronger and more flexible, and I could take more liberties when it came to my diet without worrying about gaining back weight. I was floored at the amount of inches I lost when my follow-up measurements were taken. It was unbelievable.

I have three small children and do not have time to spend hours in the gym. My workout can be done anytime, anywhere, and in about an hour. Four to five hours a week and I'm done. I recently went on vacation and was able to take my workout with me. It is fantastic. I truly believe that anyone can go on a diet and lose weight by limiting caloric intake. No matter how disciplined people are, you cannot eat like a bird forever. The fact is that the only way to keep it off and change the shape of your body is to exercise. And not just any exercise. You need to do the right exercise for you. The Exude program gives you all of that and more. I finally found the answer to my life-long struggle with my weight. Exude has changed my shape and my whole perspective on achieving and maintaining life-long health and fitness. My sincere thanks to all who have and continue to show me I CAN and I WILL escape my weight for good!!!

NAME: Ann Marie Curd-Fruhauf

DATE: May 2, 2003

AGE: 41

TOTAL INCHES LOST: 22.25

TOTAL WEIGHT LOST: 33 pounds

TIME IT TOOK TO LOSE THE WEIGHT: 9 months

PRIOR EXERCISE REGIMEN: I would go through periods when I would exercise regularly for a while but then would give up whatever I had started because I felt like I was not getting anywhere for all the time I spent in the gym. When I was on an exercise kick, I would usually spend endless hours on a treadmill or stairmaster or take some type of step class.

CURRENT EXERCISE REGIMEN: I do my prescribed Exude workout on my own 4 to 5 times a week.

PRIOR EATING HABITS: Before losing my weight, I would not be conscious of any portion sizes that I was eating. I also would often eat high fat and simple carbohydrates. I very rarely ate vegetables and fruit. That, combined with little to no exercise, caused me to consistently gain weight over the years.

CURRENT EATING HABITS: I am currently eating primarily a low-fat, complex-carbohydrate diet. I try to include all of the food groups in my daily eating. I have also begun combining my eating schedule with my workout schedule, which fuels my body more efficiently (a tip I picked up from my Exude consultant). For example, I will try and eat more carbohydrate-rich foods prior to performing my Exude program and more protein after completing my workout to promote my weight loss as well as my muscle strength and endurance. Having said that, I am able to indulge myself from time to time as the efficiency of my workouts allows me some leeway in my dietary choices.

THE MAIN FACTOR THAT HELPED ANN MARIE TO ESCAPE HER WEIGHT: Obviously, eating a more balanced, healthy diet has helped me shed pounds; however, my Exude workout is the primary reason that I am not only keeping the weight off but am reshaping my entire body. I still have more weight to lose, but this is the first time I can say that I am confident the pounds and inches will continue to drop off. Thank goodness for the Exude program.

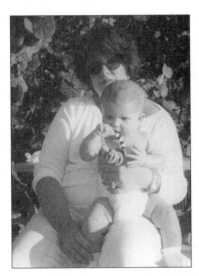 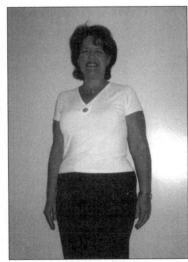

Ann Marie Curd-Fruhauf

Lori Roman—60-Plus Weight Loss

I've had a weight problem since before I started kindergarten. In fact, I was fat from preschool all the way through college and twenty years after that. Each year or two I'd try the newest fad diet. If I listed all the diets and diet programs that I'd been on from A to Z, I could get at least 50 percent of the alphabet. Let's see, to name a few: The Atkins Diet, The

Beverly Hills Diet, The Cabbage Soup Diet, The Diet Center Diet, The Grapefruit Diet, The Hilton Head Island Diet, Jenny Craig, et cetera. Do you see what I mean? I went through ten letters of the alphabet and named seven off the top of my head without even trying to think of the other diets shoved in the back of my brain. I haven't even started naming all the diet doctors that I had been to who had diets of their own. One doctor was called The Gefilte Fish Doctor because Gefilte Fish was one of the recommended foods on his diet. Needless to say, there were many.

Well, by the time I reached forty and hadn't lost the baby fat I started kindergarten with, nor the additional fifty-plus pounds that followed, I started to have aches and pains in my body that people twice my age have. I realized it was time to get serious. I knew that if I were to succeed, I needed to cover all the bases, *diet and exercise.*

I'd heard about Exude in various magazines and saw bits and pieces of an infomercial and thought to myself, *Why not? You've tried everything else.* I knew it was going to be difficult. My motto was always "I hate exercising. I'd rather not eat any food than exercise." But of course, I neither exercised nor gave up the food. That's why I was in this predicament to begin with.

Anyway, I made my first step and called Exude. I spoke with a program director who didn't seem to wince when I told him how much weight I had to lose. On my first appointment I met with Edward, who was positive and encouraging. My second visit to Exude was an eye-opening experience, to say the least. I met with Lee, who evaluated my overall physical ability, claiming she was putting me through a nonclinical fitness assessment. I went through the exercises in front of a wall of mirrors, which resembled a dance studio. I remember being so uncomfortable with the way my body looked that I couldn't stand looking at myself in the mirror. As hard as it was, I did manage to look at myself in the mirror for a few seconds at a time and so began my journey. Once Lee had evaluated my physical ability, I began meeting with my trainer three days a week. In addition to working out with him, I began my assigned homework plan and worked out two additional days a week on my own.

Lee thought I would benefit from meeting with one of Exude's nutritionists, who worked with me and my daily food intake according to my lifestyle and my specific food likes and dislikes. She recommended *a plan,* not *a diet,* that I could really stick to, including foods that were both nutritious and tasted good this way, so I did not feel deprived.

What can I say about my experience with Exude? It's been nothing short of miraculous. I've lost close to seventy-five pounds. In fact, I've lost more pounds and inches than I have with any other program that *I'd ever been on*. I've also stayed on this program longer than I have *with any other program*. In addition, I've gained a healthy lifestyle and attitude about myself. I now exercise five days a week consistently, watch what I eat without stressing over it (and am realistic about it), and feel and look years younger. Those aches and pains have disappeared, and, what's more, these changes are here to stay, not to mention the additional that will come!

NAME: Lori Roman

DATE: December 9, 2002

AGE: 42

TOTAL INCHES LOST: 35

TOTAL WEIGHT LOST: 85 pounds

TIME IT TOOK TO LOSE THE WEIGHT: 2 years

PRIOR EXERCISE REGIMEN: Very occasionally I attended water aerobics classes.

CURRENT EXERCISE REGIMEN: After meeting with Lee at Exude two years ago, I have followed my Exude program and stuck with exercising 5 days a week for at least one hour. I follow my main day program 2–3 times, which is a full-body program and then do my off-day routine on the other days, which includes more cardiovascular exercises and abdominal exercises—all on my own!

PRIOR EATING HABITS: My past eating habits and choices were not the best. I would eat too many or larger portions of carbohydrates and desserts than I should have. I didn't pay attention to portion control or size and would basically eat until I was full. I had tried everything with little or no results, sometimes gaining even more weight after all the effort I put in. I treated the weight gain and lack of exercise with quick-fix diet tricks I thought would help me to reach my goals. My weight-loss efforts include a variety of different physicians who specialize in weight loss, hypnosis, Optifast, Jenny Craig, NutriSystem, the Diet Center, and Weight Watchers. It was not only a challenge to make nutrition a consistent part of my lifestyle but even more difficult to be consistent with the proper exercise routine.

CURRENT EATING HABITS: I have changed my eating habits immensely and now incorporate healthier choices and better portion size and control. I try to be consistent with my nutrition and stay away from drastic changes or diets in general. I basically stick to eating fish 3–4 times weekly and limit my carbohydrate and fat intake. Another big change for me is that I now think about what I am eating before I just put it in my mouth, paying attention to when I feel satisfied instead of eating until I am full.

THE MAIN FACTOR THAT HELPED LORI ROMAN TO ESCAPE HER WEIGHT: Having a lot of COMMITMENT AND PERSERVERENCE is what helped me stick with my Exude program. When I eventually started seeing results and feeling better, I wanted to work even harder to achieve all of my goals. I knew I would need to be committed for a long time and know it is just part of my life.

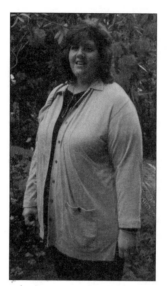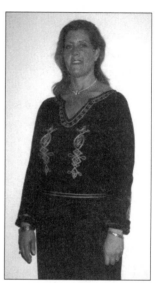

Lori Roman

Index